MW00416414

"An insightful, heartfelt, and honest look at the importance of communication in building and sustaining professional and interpersonal relationships. Dr. Nimesh H. Patel shares many life lessons learned, some the hard way, that will add significance and perspective to your understanding of the deep human need for meaningful interactions."

JAMES C. SCOGGIN JR., CEO, Methodist Health System

"After spending my entire legal career representing health care providers, this book by Dr. Nimesh H. Patel is a must-read for every medical doctor who aspires to be the best. It's a sage reminder to practitioners across the country that the practice of medicine, when extraordinary, is just as much an art as it is a science. *Extraordinary Doctor* is a succinct road map to the road less traveled in the health care profession."

JOSEPH F. CONIGLIO, managing shareholder, health care and FDA practice, Greenberg Traurig, LLP

"*Extraordinary Doctor* is an insightful and engaging chronicle of Dr. Nimesh H. Patel's journey from an ambitious young doctor to the empathetic and respected physician leader he is today. His story illustrates how, with commitment and perseverance, you can develop the emotional and self-management skills that are necessary for true personal and professional fulfillment."

JOHN F. MCCRACKEN, PhD, clinical professor of health care leadership, Naveen Jindal School of Management, University of Texas at Dallas

extraordinary
doctor

how EMOTIONAL INTELLIGENCE

drives a PHYSICIAN'S SUCCESS

———————————

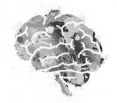

extraordinary
doctor

NIMESH H. PATEL, MD

PAGE TWO

Cataloguing in publication information is available from Library and Archives Canada.
ISBN 978-1-77458-530-6 (paperback)
ISBN 978-1-77458-532-0 (ebook)

Page Two
pagetwo.com

Edited by Scott Steedman and Kendra Ward
Copyedited by Steph VanderMeulen
Cover design by Taysia Louie and Cameron McKague
Interior design by Taysia Louie

extraordinarydoctor.com

TO MY MOM, DAD, AND BROTHER,

ASHA, HASMUKH, AND NIHAR:

*Your strength and resilience
encourage me to be extraordinary.*

TO MY WIFE, BINA:

*Your faith in us has lifted me higher than
I could imagine. Thank you for the many
unselfish weary nights helping me
express the best version of myself in this book.*

TO MY THREE DAUGHTERS,

LANA, LILA, AND LIV:

*You inspire me to be better, and
watching you grow fills my heart.*

And in loving memory of MAYA PALNITKAR.

Contents

INTRODUCTION

The Real World Is Not Medical School

F EBRUARY 23, 2003.

I heard the phone ringing at what seemed like a god-awful hour. Rubbing my eyes, I leaned over and looked at the clock.

"What the heck, it's 8:01 a.m.," I muttered to myself.

I had never slept in that late. But I was in my fourth year of medical school, and instead of taking a breezy elective rotation, I'd been taking overnight emergency calls with the neurosurgery residents. I wanted to get a jump start on my next journey. To me, that was dedication.

But I had taken the previous night off and enjoyed that liberty with my graduating medical school classmates. Work hard, play hard, right? Besides, we'd all soon be resident doctors without a life.

"Hello?" I answered the phone in a deep, groggy voice.

"Hi, Nimesh, it's Karen from the medical school admissions office. The early match results came out this morning." Pause. "I'm sorry, but you didn't match."

I swung my legs around and sat up on the edge of my bed, holding the phone, shaking my head in disbelief. "You have got to be kidding me," I said.

I didn't match anywhere. I refused to believe it. Mainly because I had religiously put in the discipline and devotion for so long. Each day, I practiced the test questions for the boards. Each morning, I went to the hospital before sunrise, and I left after sunset. This wasn't only about achieving a career goal. This was about relentless commitment and belief in myself to achieve that goal—only to fall short. My confidence was shaken. I felt nauseated.

But the reality was that it didn't matter. I did not make the cut. I had failed.

In medical school, I always felt that the students who chose surgery were a different breed. And the students who chose neurosurgery... well, we were the Spartans. I was born a Spartan and had paid my dues to earn that privilege. So I thought.

On the other end of the phone, the voice repeated the words in a regretful tone. "I'm sorry. It was a competitive year."

The silence stretched. I thanked Karen, hung up, and lay back down, hoping it was just a dream that had gone awry. But it wasn't.

I didn't have a backup plan. Why should I have even considered one? Over the next few days, I slid into a downward spiral. I was overcome with feelings of doom. I could hardly function. I refused to celebrate with anyone else who had matched into a residency program, because I could not bear to tell them that I had failed. I sure didn't want anyone's pity.

At the end of the week, I mustered up the last hope left inside me. I called every neurosurgery program where I felt I had interviewed well. Everyone responded in the same way: "I'm sorry. You were our runner-up." The words hurt, but I kept dialing the numbers, hearing "sorry" over and over again.

Most program directors were polite, but a few were a bit more direct. One director even told me that I should consider another field in medicine, implying that I did not have the capabilities for neurosurgery. Humiliated, I picked up the phone again. I couldn't bring myself to accept that all my work was not good enough.

My very last call, one I almost didn't make, went through. I knew what I wanted to say to Dr. Kelvin Von Roenn, the program director for the highly reputable RUSH University Neurosurgery in Chicago.

"If you give me a chance, I will work hard for you and make you proud," I told him. "If you're hiring someone who knows how to take tests, I could do a better job of that. And if you're hiring someone who will work hard, be a strong contributor to the organization, and who is willing to learn, then I'd like for you to consider hiring me."

Against all odds, I heard, "OK, let's talk some more."

My world shifted with those words.

SIX YEARS LATER, I found myself as the co-chief resident of RUSH's neurosurgery program. I sat in Von Roenn's office during his smoke break. He was a stoic man, tough on the outside and gentle on the inside, depending on the day. We referred to him plainly as "Von Roenn," which was always spoken with reverence.

A stack of files sat on his desk. Every file represented a neurosurgery applicant interviewing for a job. Each file held someone's dream. They wouldn't all make it.

With a cigarette in hand, Von Roenn flipped open the closest file. "Remember when you were interviewing for this program?" he asked me.

"I do," I said. Even six years later, the question made me feel uneasy.

Von Roenn must have seen my embarrassment when my smile quickly faded and I looked down, because he let go of the file and pointed his finger at me.

"At the level we're interviewing, each one of you is an all-star on paper. I took the chance on you because, one, I felt sorry for you," he said gruffly, with a smirk. "But two, and more importantly, the day you called, I heard that sincerity in your voice and knew you'd be a good resident. I followed my gut, and I'm glad I did."

His big caterpillar mustache turned up in a broad smile. "It took a lot of heart to give us that call. Surely you don't think you're the only special one in the world who's needed to pick themselves off the ground to get what they want?"

"What?" I said, surprised. Could it be that I wasn't the only one with a deeply buried secret of failure?

Von Roenn continued. "Listen, if you want to be successful as a neurosurgeon, we have you covered. But more importantly, if you want to be a highly successful physician, you need to know how to operate both inside and outside the operating room."

He gestured to a second stack of files, cigarette smoke trailing his hand as he did. "This group here? They have stellar scores, but they don't understand the first thing about people. You understand people. I could tell that from the way you spoke when you called me—you didn't just have guts, you had empathy. That's why I gave you a chance."

The Real World

The real world is different from medical school.

As medical students, we train for years taking tests. We become proficient at memorizing checklists and mnemonics. Then, as young resident physicians, we dedicate years to learning how to diagnose and treat patients. All these skill sets are crucial to our long-term success in clinical medicine. However, to be highly successful and fulfilled as a physician in the dynamic world of clinics and hospitals demands a distinct set of skills, and that is not even *part* of our medical training.

The disparity between what we're taught and what is expected of us in the real world isn't rooted in theory, fortunately. The real world requires emotional intelligence—that is, self-awareness and communication skills that allow us to optimize our performance while building trust and alliances. Simply put, there is a serious gap in our physician development.

As a weary yet proud medical student or resident, you will feel inundated with medical information, as if you are drinking from a fire hydrant. You aspire to exude credibility, confidence, and trustworthiness. And secretly, you desire to be a charismatic physician known for your effortless charm, bedside manner, and sharp intellect. But you're uncertain how to acquire the necessary skills to become that person. I know this because I used to be you. That's why I wrote this book.

The hidden skills and insights required to bridge the gap between being an ordinary physician, regardless of clinical proficiency, and a highly successful and fulfilled physician are grounded in real-world experience. And all are found in the pages of this book.

The Research

As a physician by profession and a pragmatist by personality, I wanted to ensure my advice was as unbiased as possible. I conducted qualitative research. I dedicated countless hours to having conversations with medical professionals, psychologists, and malpractice attorneys. I sat with nurses across various clinical settings, including clinics, intensive care units (ICUs), and hospital floors. I stood in front of hospital administrators to gain insight into their priorities for young physicians. I sought input from my business school professors to analyze ways to enhance economics and patient value in health care. Fortunately, none of them were shy.

Lastly, I spoke with residents and medical students. What nonclinical questions were most pressing? What did they wish someone was teaching them? I also dug deep into my memories of being a new doctor. What had I most needed to know at key moments in my career?

I wanted to get this book right.

What I learned I have curated for you in the pages that follow. You will discover:

- **Chapter 1:** Why people skills are the greatest complement to your clinical expertise

- **Chapter 2:** How to distinguish yourself in the real world outside medical school

- **Chapter 3:** Why clinical skills are never enough to make you an extraordinary physician

- **Chapter 4:** Why knowing yourself is the best return on your investment

- **Chapter 5:** How to confidently handle seven tricky scenarios you're likely to encounter

- **Chapter 6:** How to optimize your performance by understanding your motivation—including its dark side

- **Chapter 7:** How to forward your career in medicine through building strategic alliances

- **Chapter 8:** How to enhance patient care through subtle verbal and nonverbal techniques

- **Chapter 9:** Why specific actions and words not taught in medical school will give you an advantage for the rest of your career

- **Chapter 10:** How to harness the soft power of empathy

- **Chapter 11:** How to master the art of strategic silence

If you want to be both extraordinary and fulfilled as a physician—with more control over your career and more opportunities—this book will help you develop the emotional intelligence to make that happen.

This book is the one I wish I'd had as a young physician to show me how to succeed in medicine in the long term. It is my apologia for the belief that emotional intelligence is an essential skill that drives a doctor's success.

That day in Von Roenn's smoke-filled office, he gave me a tremendous gift of self-redemption. Six years prior, during my desperate phone calls, I had been grappling with self-doubt, seeking validation externally. The truth was that I had accomplished that task for everyone else, but not for myself. In that moment, Von Roenn's affirmations restored my faith in myself. He helped me rediscover the trust I had lost in myself after the dreadful news of not matching. Because of him, now, twenty years later, I am inspired to never abandon myself and to continue to practice resilience, even if the obstacles seem impossible to overcome.

From adapting to diverse personalities to appreciating the worth of every individual and dollar in my immigrant parents' small-town business, I learned invaluable lessons that have shaped me. These experiences instilled in me humility and the dedication to hard work, traits that became indispensable during my journey through medical school and neurosurgery residency.

The intense drive to succeed stems from multiple isolated experiences from my childhood. The anguish of nearly missing out on a neurosurgery residency all those years ago remains a defining moment that shaped the trajectory of my career. Today, as the section chief of Neurosurgery and executive medical director at the Methodist Health System in

Dallas, and as the managing partner of a private investment fund, I am reminded of the truth—that my journey was fueled by the choice to seek reconsideration from multiple neurosurgery programs. Failure became the catalyst for my success. Dr. Von Roenn passed away a few months after our conversation. His resident teaching award sitting on my desk is a poignant reminder of his wisdom. That day in his office, I vowed to be more than an ordinary physician: I would be a highly successful and fulfilled physician. An extraordinary doctor. I believe you can be too.

1

People Skills Are a Key to Success

———

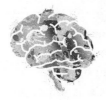

WHEN I was in my third year in medical school, I witnessed one of the most astonishing scenes I've ever seen in a hospital and got my first hint that there might be more to being a doctor than what I was taught in class.

As an avid fan of TV shows about doctors, I believed I had a good grasp of what occurred within hospital walls. I anticipated meeting the fast-paced heroic surgeon, the tireless resident, and the compassionate pediatrician caring for the sick but stoic child. However, my expectations were shattered during one of my initial rotations in a pediatric ICU.

Walking into a room, I encountered a distressing scene: a father verbally steamrolling a pediatric oncologist. The doctor had been explaining the side effects of the radiation being administered to the man's eight-year-old daughter, Emily, who was battling a pontine glioma, a highly aggressive brain tumor with no known cure.

"Just stop, stop right there," the father said, his voice trembling with distress. "Can't you do something more to help her with her pain?" He rose from his seat. "All you do is wake her up all hours of the night, stab her with these needles, and give her this poison." Suddenly, he put his hands up and started shouting. "Do you even really care!? Forget it. Where's the head of Children's? I want to know my daughter is getting the best care!"

The ICU attending happened to overhear this exchange. She entered the room and, in a calm, kindly voice, said, "Hi, I'm Dr. Robinson. How can I help?"

The father turned on her and went on a fifteen-minute tirade, complaining about everything and nothing, from the side effects of the radiation to the price of the coffee. People stopped in the halls to listen, and he kept venting his frustration. The nurses, other parents, the oncologist, and I all stood back in shocked silence, watching the event unfold.

Standing in my brand-new white coat, a stethoscope draped around my neck and my pockets stuffed with papers, I was glued to the scene along with everyone else. I had no idea what I would do in Dr. Robinson's role, but I assumed she was feeling threatened and defensive. I certainly was. (It turned out she wasn't, for reasons I later understood.) I noticed her leaning in, speaking in a hushed tone over the father's outburst.

Then, out of nowhere, the man became quiet and slumped back into his chair.

Dr. Robinson waited patiently and calmly, as she had been doing for a quarter of an hour. The father wiped his eyes and looked up at her. She then acknowledged his pain and frustration and proceeded to guide him through Emily's expected treatment course.

In moments such as these, when the patient outcome eludes our control despite our clinical expertise, we as physicians need to grasp who the person in front of us is. We are never merely addressing a patient or a family member. We are speaking to a father or mother, a protector and provider. This is not solely about reciting medical literature, stating facts, or detailing side effects. *It's about acknowledging and establishing connections with the various identities and roles that define the patient or their family member beyond their medical condition.*

Later that morning, I found Dr. Robinson at the nurses' station, finishing her notes. Curious, I asked about her interaction with the father. She explained that she believed the father's flare-up hadn't really been about treatment or side effects. Rather, these were a proxy for a deeper need, that of a genuine sense of understanding and empathy.

The man was at his wits' end, Dr. Robinson explained. He needed to express his frustration and helplessness in witnessing his beloved daughter sick and weak in a hospital bed, her head bald from the radiation therapy. The dam had finally burst. He simply needed to yell, emote, and release months of pent-up emotions. His demands were not personal— they had nothing to do with the oncologist, Dr. Robinson, or me, for that matter. They were a last, desperate resort, a cry for help.

You are more than
just a physician;
you also serve
as a counselor.

In that critical moment, Dr. Robinson did not confront him or refute his accusations. Instead, she acknowledged his distress, recognizing him not as an irate family member but as a concerned and helpless father. Her response—"You're a good father. I know you are in pain"—was her way of seeing beyond the surface and connecting with the man's emotional turmoil. It was a choice to take the high road, showing empathy and understanding in a difficult situation.

After his outburst, the father calmed down and continued to be a vigilant participant in Emily's care. The young girl valiantly battled the cancer until it was time to move on from her father's arms. When she did, she was surrounded by family and the medical team at the hospital, who had formed close bonds with her because of her courageous spirit.

You are more than just a physician; you also serve as a counselor. While you may know the medical diagnosis, aiding a family in coping is equally your responsibility. Dr. Robinson could not save Emily, but she could provide comfort and psychological safety by recognizing that Emily's father was suffering as well.

Although this skill set isn't explicitly taught, it is one our patients and their families expect of us. Mastery of these skills will transform you from an ordinary doctor into an extraordinary doctor.

Focus On the Big Picture

Patient information often arrives fragmented, resembling pieces of a puzzle. Your role is to assemble these pieces, discerning the larger picture by understanding your patients' true intentions.

Families in medical settings may struggle to articulate fear and emotional pain, often suppressing these feelings until they reach a breaking point. Similar to a pressure cooker without a safety valve, emotions can erupt unexpectedly. To avert such outbursts, adept physicians gauge the emotional temperature of the room. How are the patient and their family coping?

When tension is palpable in the room, initiate a conversation that acknowledges the prevailing emotions. Use phrases such as "I understand that this is a challenging situation. Share with me what's happening. What are your thoughts?" Proactively inviting discussion and genuinely listening allows families to release pent-up emotions before they escalate.

If emotions do erupt, be Dr. Robinson. Stay silent and let the person express their distress or guilt. Resist the urge to retaliate. The white coat serves as a shield, enabling us to stand firm. If we maintain composure and refrain from taking the storm personally, our empathetic silence can allow intense emotions to dissipate.

Thinking back now, I suspect that the pediatric oncologist missed the big picture. Rather than focusing solely on the child's symptoms, he could have posed more comprehensive questions to the father, the answers of which would have provided the additional puzzle pieces to complete the picture:

- "How are you doing?"
- "How have things been going?"
- "Have things become better or worse?"
- "What are you doing to take care of yourself?"

There are two strategies for finding the missing puzzle pieces: avoiding fixation on superficial details, and identifying the patient's true problem.

Don't Fixate On Superficial Details

That father exemplified what many patients and families often do. He did not directly discuss a deeper issue but rather channeled his anxiety into specific questions instead, those about causes, symptoms, medication doses, and side effects.

When he complained about not getting the best care, his actual concern was his guilt and helplessness. Since he couldn't ease Emily's nausea and vomiting, he focused on enhancing her nutrition to alleviate her suffering. The surface issues were nutrition and radiation side effects (the girl losing her hair), but the deeper issue was his grief.

The oncologist could have leaned forward and asked, "How are you doing?" That might have eased some of the tension and the father might not have lost his temper.

Most cases are not as simple as "My elbow hurts," a situation where we can solve everything by treating the elbow. That visit is straightforward and rare. We are in the business of identifying symptoms and treating diseases. To treat the medical issue, we must be willing to consider the big picture, and the whole patient.

Identify the Patient's True Problem

Every patient issue has three aspects: physiological, psychological, and unknown.

Many patients come to the doctor asking for help with at least two of these aspects. In response, 90 percent of the time, most physicians address only the *physiological* problem.

Physicians are trained to handle the physiological. Anatomy, chemistry, data, and statistics do not faze us. We suggest solutions for patients easily. In contrast, when presented with problems that are mainly psychological in nature, we struggle. We have not been trained to communicate with patients in emotional pain, or to address psychological causes for physiological issues. We lack the skills to determine what is most important to the patient.

When working with a patient or their family, also look for the *psychological* part of the problem. Allow the patient to tell you the impact of the issue on their emotions. The doctor could have asked the father:

- "What do you think about what I said?"
- "How well are you coping with this situation?"

And then the doctor could have simply listened.

Lastly, do not gloss over the *unknown piece*. Medicine as a whole may not yet have an answer, and admitting to the unknown is stressful. Good patient care means explaining the boundaries of what is known without seeming ill prepared. The job requires delivering the unknown gracefully—which means facing up to our limitations and the limitations of medicine as it stands today.

Every patient issue
has three aspects:
physiological,
psychological,
and unknown.

Most areas of medicine, including cancer care, have advanced significantly in the last few decades. But we still don't really understand the root causes of many illnesses and often can't cure them. In my field, glioblastoma multiforme, an incredibly elusive brain cancer, has taken the lives of many people I care about—patients, family, and friends. Even after the surgeries, I feel helpless, knowing the disease is relentless and will take their lives within a year. I've looked into unconventional treatments everywhere because it's clear that our current knowledge falls short. The truth is, we don't know enough yet.

Admitting this to your patients is not a sign of weakness; it's being humble. The humility of acknowledging the unknown builds trust, the essential foundation of any doctor-patient relationship.

The oncologist could have said one of the following to the heartbroken father:

- "Let's talk about what we know and what we don't know."

- "Truth be told, science is always evolving. If a plant-based diet doesn't cause harm, I don't see any reason why you can't try it."

Good patient care from a big-picture perspective means connecting with the patient at a level deeper than a checklist.

Emotional Intelligence Fills the Gap

High-performing people often become fixated solely on clinical outcomes. I, too, used to fall into that trap. Developing excellence takes an intense time commitment. And time is a limited resource. We prioritize our commitment to the mastery of certain skills at the cost of neglecting others. The oversights compound.

Physicians also frequently judge other physicians based solely on clinical skills, which is an incomplete measure. The mere ability to diagnose a patient, give orders to a nurse, or know how to take out a brain tumor isn't proof of success.

It may come as a surprise that medical school and residency teach only *half* of what we need to be highly successful and fulfilled as physicians. Yes, clinical skills are critical, but the other half of what we need to know is just as important—yet we can traverse our entire careers without formal instruction in the fundamental qualities that ultimately define the physician we seek to become.

The other half of the critical skills are *people skills*, often referred to as emotional intelligence (EQ). This includes how to establish authority and influence through effective communication, empathy, and self-awareness. Developing emotional intelligence will set you apart from the rest of your colleagues.

Doctors who master EQ will excel, while those who don't will stagnate. The enlightened physicians earn influence and opportunities that would otherwise never be available. They also learn to become better leaders by building alliances and high-functioning teams. Meanwhile, the doctors who refuse to learn these skills struggle with dissatisfaction and isolation throughout their careers.

Please understand: physicians who focus only on clinical skills can indeed have a thriving and successful practice. However, achieving both success and fulfillment demands more. It requires both clinical expertise *and* people skills. It involves cultivating alliances and mastering the art of bringing out the best in both your colleagues and yourself.

It also demands hard work, but if you have made it through medical school, then I know you're already accustomed to hard work. Why invest so much effort, sacrifice so greatly, only to settle for less than your full potential? In the pages ahead, you'll discover the framework to ensure your hard work pays off.

Our greatest limitation is the ceiling we impose on ourselves. Instead of hitting up against that ceiling, learn to raise it. Develop the people skills you'll need to take control of your career. Rise to your full potential. After all, you always have.

You are a high achiever and therefore no stranger to the challenges of change. The ability to listen and adapt has been your strength and has separated you from the rest of your colleagues. Now let me complement your innate and well-earned success with the people skills to be extraordinary.

Doctor, distinguish yourself in the real world.

2

How to Operate in the Real World

———

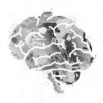

MEET ME in the hallway outside Operating Room 22. Make sure you're wearing a surgical cap and a mask. Go ahead, push open the operating room doors. Look over to the left—you can see me standing over the patient, Mr. Donahue, in a flexed and focused posture. Listen closely… that's his heartbeat coming from the anesthesia machine. *Beep. Beep. Beep.*

I'm dotting the few remaining drops of blood in Mr. Donahue's nose with a piece of cotton. Eric Clapton is playing over the ceiling speakers. After three hours of work on a high-risk brain surgery through the nose, I feel accomplished. Job done.

Brain surgery through the nose is complex enough. But surgery on a softball-sized tumor touching the carotid artery, one of the major arteries of the brain, is exceptionally risky.

If I push or pull on the tumor, it could move the wrong way, and catastrophic complications could quickly follow.

Fortunately, everything went according to plan today. I removed the tumor without a hitch. We're just starting to close the access to the brain from the nose. My body begins to relax.

Dabbing the spots of blood is a routine cleanup. But today, the dots suddenly turn into a small trickle. *That's odd*, I think to myself. I hold pressure again, feeling a little annoyed because this unexpected bleeding will delay the rest of my day. But no big deal; the pressure should resolve the issue soon.

There's an old surgical proverb: "All bleeding eventually stops. Either it stops, or you run out of blood." We surgeons have a morbid sense of humor.

I remove the pressure from the cottonoid, and to my surprise, the trickle of blood continues. My minor annoyance turns into dismay. I turn to my steadfast nurse practitioner, Stacey, to get a bit of emotional support when, in the blink of an eye, blood explodes through Mr. Donahue's nose. The flow is so furious that blood is soon frothing out of his mouth. I rapidly unroll gauze and pack it into Mr. Donahue's nose and mouth. But the blood keeps flowing, out of his mouth and up the scarlet-red gauze so quickly that it's soon dripping onto my boots.

Stacey and I look at each other. We are both thinking the same thing: *This guy is going to bleed out on the table.*

"This is not good," I mumble to myself, remaining unemotional and composed. My neurosurgery colleague, Dr. Stewart, scrubs out without saying a word. He picks up the phone on the back wall and calls to ready the angiogram suite. The operating room team starts lifesaving measures on the body in front of me.

The smooth voice of Eric Clapton turns into an alarming "Code Blue OR 22, Code Blue OR 22, Code Blue OR 22."

The doors fly open; people rush into the room. The anesthesiologist rips down the sterile field and squeezes the bag of IV fluids.

I am in lifesaving mode, focused and detached. The possible actionable scenarios fill my head, one after the other. I've visited this safe place many times over the last two decades. But my experience tells me that in this case, today, it won't matter. Mr. Donahue is going to die. He is going to bleed his life away on my operating room table. My heart drops into my stomach.

As we enter the angiography suite, in the intensity of this life-threatening moment, my inner stoic acknowledges the gravity of the situation.

"This is not going well," I say. "What are we thinking here?" It is my humble way of asking for help without feeling embarrassed or vulnerable.

Dr. Stewart stretches out Mr. Donahue's arm and, with pinpoint precision, threads a catheter through his wrist and up to his brain. He then shoots a dye to map out all the blood vessels of the brain.

"Where's the leak?" I ask him. With each passing second, more blood is pooling on the floor.

"There, the petrous carotid artery."

As neurosurgeons, we know this blood vessel sits in an area of the skull that is nearly impossible to reach safely or rapidly. This man is going to die, or he is going to have a

The *content* of the information is not as important as the *delivery*.

massive cerebral hemispheric stroke. Either way, there is no favorable scenario.

Where did I go wrong? Where was my mistake? I stand there, stuck for one long moment in guilt.

"We were nowhere near there," Dr. Stewart says, pointing to the leak and then to where we operated. "There was no reason for it to tear."

Five minutes later, I am making my way to the waiting room. I am jittery, nauseated; my hands are clammy. Mr. Donahue's daughter has no idea that I am about to turn her world upside down with the news.

I sit next to her in the waiting room. I steady my breathing, the same way I do before placing a clip across a brain aneurysm.

Speak slowly.

I walk Mr. Donahue's daughter through what happened. I explain that it was unpredictable and we have temporary control of the situation. Then I tell her the two most likely outcomes: her father will die or suffer a massive cerebral hemispheric stroke.

As I imagined, the truth hits her hard; she is stunned and then starts to sob.

"What does this mean?" she asks, her voice broken by despair.

I am careful to be unemotional, direct, and factual with my answers, no matter the outcome. And then I wait. A few more clear and concise facts about the next steps. I feel she needs to know everything. The more nervous I am, the more clinical and factual I become.

She nods her head as if she understands, but her eyes are somewhere else. She is overwhelmed. I am not connecting with her. Emotionally, she is barely hanging on. If anything, I am making her more anxious.

Ironically, in my sincere effort to be truly transparent, the speed and quantity of information I gave her have made her even more apprehensive. She has dropped into what I call "emotional survival mode," and now she needs me to be competent by another measure.

In that split second, I realize that no matter how precarious the situation, the *content* of the information is not as important as the *delivery*. And that is one thing we are not taught in medical school. The *feel* of the conversation.

A successful surgeon must maintain composure under pressure, and that comes at the price of tucking away their emotions. It takes me a moment to find mine. I face Mr. Donahue's daughter, making sure our eyes are on the same level. After a pause to steady my energy, I start speaking in a slow, measured cadence, guiding her through what I know and don't know and what we plan on doing next.

Striking the right balance between confidence and compassion, modesty and trustworthiness is crucial. Personally, I've noticed that when I'm stressed, I tend to speak too quickly, so I make a conscious effort to maintain an even, considered tone. I conclude by saying, "I reassure you, we will do everything possible to save him." After another pause, I stand up and walk away.

BACK IN the angiography suite, I rejoin the team, who are in a huddle. Dr. Stewart has seen this situation before and is first to speak. He proposes what is basically a neurosurgery Hail Mary, a crazy idea that might just work. It might also make things worse. No medical textbook covers this situation. We nod and go straight to work.

The first attempt to seal off the bleeding was not effective. We now have to *sacrifice* the left carotid artery. We have decided that potentially killing Mr. Donahue's ability to speak and understand language is a burden we are ready to carry if it means he can live. People's brain structures vary, and his may put him at risk of some catastrophic consequences, or not—we just don't have the time to test it. The only way to find out is to try it.

Dr. Stewart places the coils into the left carotid artery to kill it off.

We hold our breath.

Slowly, both sides of the brain fill from only one carotid artery.

We finally breathe.

The Hail Mary worked.

I INCLUDE this story to point to two critical truths that are not taught in medical school:

1 You need to *earn* your patient's trust in a heartbeat.
2 Asking for help is a sign of maturity, not incompetence.

These are two unspoken and readily expected skills in the work environment. Real-world success requires not just technical skill but also new ways of thinking. The emotionally intelligent physician knows how to earn the trust of patients and families and listens to and works with, not against, their whole health care team.

You Need to *Earn* Your Patient's
Trust in a Heartbeat

When we encounter patients and their families, they are often having one of the worst days of their lives. They are in what I previously mentioned as "emotional survival mode." These patients and families feel helpless and are looking for reassurance. If your verbal and nonverbal communication does not invite trust in a way they expect, they will lose confidence in your abilities and start to second-guess your decision-making.

The key to earning trust is deceptively simple yet challenging to master. Emotionally intelligent communication goes beyond the clarity and honesty emphasized in medical school, and it can serve as a lifeline to both patients and their families.

If Mr. Donahue's daughter had lost trust in the surgical team (or in me, the team's representative), her doubt and fear and the myriad associated questions would have consumed valuable time, a luxury her father could not afford. Such a loss of trust could have seriously reduced his chances of survival.

Medical schools do not teach young doctors how to earn their patients' trust. Yet every interaction hinges on this skill. Trust is a continuous exchange of transparency between people. When you wear the white coat, trust is automatically *loaned* to you. However, patients and families can easily repossess that trust. To have trust *given* to you, you must earn it.

Patients gauge us primarily through one critical metric: trust. It's not just what we say but also how we say it. While

Medical schools do not teach young doctors how to earn their patients' trust.

competencies such as formulating a differential diagnosis or selecting the best treatment plan are important, trust surpasses them all. The pivotal elements are people skills, including being able to communicate with emotional intelligence and knowing how to listen attentively rather than delivering a lecture to the patient. As I said, you didn't learn those skills in medical school, but you'll need them every day if you want to get ahead.

Asking for Help Is a Sign of Maturity, Not Incompetence

If I hadn't asked for help, Mr. Donahue would have died.

Without the quick thinking of our anesthesiologist and the collaborative efforts of the operating room team, along with my neurosurgery colleague, Dr. Stewart, Mr. Donahue's fate that day could have been dire. Dr. Stewart, being an expert in endovascular neurosurgery, proposed the innovative idea of sacrificing the left carotid artery, which ultimately proved successful. My experience underscores the significance of collaborative practices and a willingness to seek input even when one possesses the expertise.

Because of its unexpected outcome, the case was examined by a peer review committee. I was taken aback by the comments provided. One remark stood out: that the act of seeking help, specifically from another expert, "showcased maturity in recognizing the value of collective wisdom and expertise."

It stands to reason that failing to ask for help when it's needed is an immature professional judgment. I am confident during life-threatening circumstances, but having an experienced team provides a vital counterbalance in an emotionally tense situation. They function as a second head, thinking clearly and looking at every obstacle from several unique angles. I feel more secure and focused with them supporting and helping me and each other. Not having their guidance would have meant failure in this case—and in many other cases.

High-risk operations are common. I've learned that even the very best surgeons know when to ask for help. That is the exact opposite of how we are trained to practice in medical school, but it is a highly effective strategy. Physicians build their careers by competing to be the best. In medical school, it was all about individual achievements, not teamwork, at least academically. Never mind leaning on someone else with similar strengths or who was better than I was at a particular task. I didn't want to be embarrassed. I didn't want to come across as inadequate, so I went at it alone. Back then, I could rely only on myself to get the job done.

It wasn't until I began my practice that I realized the importance of involving others. Instead of viewing health care professionals around me as threats—not just fellow neurosurgeons or other specialists but also nurses, medical assistants, and administrators—I enlisted their help. It is not a competition. It is a collective effort, where we come together for our patients and our preservation. When we do, everyone wins.

Let me show you not just how to ask for help but how to do it with emotional intelligence.

3

Clinical Skills Are Never Enough

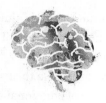

ONE WEEKEND, I was consulted on two challenging cases, each presenting its own complexities. One patient was a seventy-year-old retired librarian, and the other was a forty-nine-year-old social worker. Diagnosing and treating their conditions wasn't particularly difficult. But I found myself struggling with the question of what value I could offer these patients and their families in seemingly unwinnable situations.

Sunday was a dark and somber morning. I walked down the long hospital corridor, lost in thought, staring at the glossy floor tiles reflecting the harsh glow of the florescent lights above. I thought to myself, *I've done more brain biopsies in my career than I care to remember, and still always dread seeing the telltale pattern of glioblastoma multiforme.*

The outcome of this brain cancer is almost always the same: the patient will be dead within a year. That day, I was scheduled to take care of two more.

When I started my career, the thrills and complexities of each case gave me a sense of emotional satisfaction. But now, after over fifteen years in the field, things feel different. I still do my job well—better, even—but the emotions have shifted from being about science and sympathizing to something more powerful.

So, I asked myself that morning, *What is the job?* Yes, it was still about being precise and skilled in surgeries, saving lives. But I couldn't help but wonder about the actual impact of my work when the result was often so grim.

Then the answer hit me. Even if it's just for a moment, I try to offer understanding to my patients. I may not be able to save them with my hands, but I will always try to save them with my heart.

That's a purpose with power. The power to make an ordinary doctor extraordinary.

I share my thoughts because the journey of understanding oneself and staying humble during challenges, whether psychological or clinical, lasts a lifetime.

Find Humility before You Are Humiliated

Back in 2003, after convincing Dr. Von Roenn to give me a chance, I was a young, proud, new resident at RUSH University in Chicago, Illinois, on my general surgery rotation. Near the end of my day, Dr. Joshua, the senior resident, called me from the operating room. "Mr. Stevens is throwing up, and I can't get away. Go check him out and see if he needs an NG tube."

"No problem," I said. I was psyched.

The previous night, Mr. Stevens had been admitted to the hospital for acute back pain and was given narcotics to control the pain. The medication works just fine, but it has known side effects. One key side effect is that narcotics cause the intestines to fall asleep. This is called an *ileus*.

Mr. Stevens's case was an excellent example of that problem. He ate and drank, but instead of the food and liquids passing through the system normally, they came right back up. He had vomited the entire night and was clearly miserable.

As I arrived, I saw the nurse in the room helping Mr. Stevens get comfortable. It was evident by his ability to confidently comfort Mr. Stevens that this nurse had been in the business a long time.

At this point in my life, I was a bit too confident and felt that I could handle anything. After all, I was now a neurosurgery Spartan-in-training. I swaggered forward with just a touch of bravado. Instead of asking the nurse for help, I confidently requested the supplies. The nurse brought me the NG tube, and I took it out of its package, curling the end of it as I had seen the one and only time I had observed the procedure. I smiled at the nurse. I was about to impress him.

I took the tube in one hand and tilted Mr. Stevens's head back with the other. Gently, I slipped the curved tip of the tube to the back of his nose. After a little tickle to his nose, the NG tube started advancing. A rush of excitement and accomplishment coursed through me. The tube was moving—I was getting it right. I thought to myself, *Not so bad! I'm good at this.*

But then Mr. Stevens started to cough. The cough turned into a gag. My eyes widened. The nurse abruptly stepped to the side. Before I could put together what was happening, Mr. Stevens projectile vomited all over my oversized scrubs and my new long white coat.

I jumped back, grimacing in disgust, and my prescription pad fell into the mess. My newly scuffed clogs were now covered in glistening emesis. The NG tube lay forlornly on the floor. I was shocked. The nurse was clearly enjoying it all.

Coincidentally, Dr. Joshua happened to appear at the door just at that moment. Unaware of or indifferent to the situation, he said to the nurse, "I need help with the patient in 326."

Before leaving with the senior resident, the nurse paused and looked me in the eye. With his eyebrow raised and his head cocked forward, he said, chuckling, "Next time, tell the patient to swallow when you advance the NG tube." His tone made it clear that he thought I was an idiot. He was right, but not for the reasons I assumed at the time.

Lacking the skill was not the issue. No one expects an eager new surgical resident to know everything. Dr. Joshua did not expect me to know how to place the NG tube; neither did the nurse. All I had to do was admit it—a big issue for young doctors—and not behave so cavalierly. The nurse would have happily helped me. Instead, I chose to flex the skills I didn't have and proved myself a fool.

A physician who presumes to know it all and does not ask questions is a fool. That physician readily takes risks with patients' lives. They are in dangerous waters.

I received a valuable lesson in this principle, along with the vomit. Unfortunately, I also portrayed myself as incompetent, which impacted how I was treated on the floor for weeks afterward.

When you lose trust, you lose influence with the patient and everyone else involved in taking care of them. It's a long road to regain that lost trust, so it is prudent to ask for help and prove yourself trustworthy from the beginning. Bottom line: when you need to admit ignorance, do it with humility and respect. Keep your pride by asking emotionally intelligent questions—for some suggestions, see below—and then, if necessary, ask for help. You will be amazed: people in health care want to help and will gladly pass on their skills and education. They will also develop a fondness for you.

You will be humbled one way or the other. The emotionally intelligent physician is in control of how that goes down.

The Good, the Bad, and the Ugly

At every point in your life, there will be someone who knows more than you. Early in your career, that person may be someone you routinely overlook: a medical assistant, a patient care technician, or the clerk who has been at the clinic or hospital for years. These people may not be at the top of the medical hierarchy, but they work with the patients every day and know what we physicians don't. Take advantage of their experience.

In the scenario above, a savvy way to admit my limitations and still feel competent would have been to ask, *"Would you mind* helping me place the NG tube?" A straightforward

A physician
who presumes to
know it all and
does not ask
questions is a fool.

statement such as that would have showcased insight to the seasoned nurse. "Would you mind?" says that I am cautious, humble, and above all, respectful of the situation. These are all things practiced individuals want to see before they give us their trust.

There will also be times when you are just not experienced enough and simply have no answer for a scenario. When ignorance of the situation inevitably happens, saying (or even just thinking) "I don't know, but I'll find out" and then subtly leaning over to the nurse or patient care technician and whispering "What do you think?" will help you establish or regain trust without diminishing your work ethic. It will set you apart from the rest.

The resident who is willing to learn will be rewarded more than the overconfident one with vomit on his shoes.

Two emotionally intelligent statements that will help you establish trust or regain trust are:

- "Would you mind...?"
- "I don't know, but I'll find out."

Why Clinical Skills Are Never Enough

The day I started my second year in residency, I met the chief resident of general surgery, Dr. Franklin, at the famous Cook County Hospital in Chicago, Illinois. Dr. Franklin was articulate, well respected, and reputably phenomenal in the operating room. The instant I met him, I was in awe of him. I wanted to be him.

Over time, though, as I became more comfortable with my new daily doctor tasks, I began to notice chinks in Dr. Franklin's armor.

Dr. Franklin had trouble getting along with certain individuals. He regularly butted heads with authority—especially the heads of nursing and other medical specialties. At times, I watched him stare at and physically confront consulting physicians, asking, "And what's the point of this consult?" His arrogant manner created an uncomfortable environment between physician colleagues.

One time, while on rounds, a proactive rotating medical intern asked a few basic questions about a patient Dr. Franklin needed to book for surgery. Dr. Franklin responded with an apathetic "Figure it out" and walked off. He was dismissive and subtly degrading, talking down to people and acting as if he knew it all. To be clear, Dr. Franklin didn't ever lose his cool, and he was never emotional or irrational. But no one enjoys being belittled.

Over time, when I had details to report to Dr. Franklin, I learned to brace myself before I called him. I also prepared myself to expect condescending words. Unfortunately, I wasn't the only target. Dr. Franklin treated everyone on the floor equally. In my eyes, the guy who had once been a star soon lost his shine.

As I started to better understand Dr. Franklin, I saw that he treated many of us as if we were working *for* him instead of *with* him. He had sharp elbows. As he became increasingly demeaning, I saw my colleagues and other medical staff quietly rebel. Clinical details dropped. Labs and scans were regarded as optional. Pages were not answered. Many of us worried that his behavior would affect patient care.

As his behavior began to cause forced errors, Dr. Franklin felt each error was a personal attack on him. He became increasingly frustrated, and the verbal punishment started to roll downhill to us junior doctors. Eventually, he unraveled from the pressure and was removed from the service for a psychological evaluation and mandatory counseling.

Similar to many physicians, Dr. Franklin was great with execution, both in operating with technical finesse and in running the service. But his great clinical skills were not enough to save him from himself. His dreadful people skills let him down.

No doctor should follow in Dr. Franklin's footsteps. Our behaviors are shaped by observing our resident colleagues and attendings: the good, the bad, and the ugly. And those bad and ugly behaviors, such as sarcasm and belittling colleagues and supporting staff, are often unconsciously absorbed during our training.

Is Everything OK?

Early in my career, while scrubbing at the sink before a surgical case, a colleague turned to me and said, "Nimesh, you're great with patients and the staff enjoys working with you. What happened today between you and the charge nurse to make you upset? The way you talked down to her seemed completely out of character. *Is everything OK?*"

In that moment, I realized that my sarcastic behavior was not typical of what was expected of me. *Is everything OK?* gently implied my comments were not acceptable. I felt embarrassed, and memories of Dr. Franklin came flooding back.

The operating room is a tense place. People, especially doctors, often relieve the tension with wild, crude, or off-color comments. It's a learned behavior, one I witnessed many times when I was a resident, working with surgeons such as Dr. Franklin, and even found myself repeating as I moved forward in my career.

But it's never OK to be sarcastic or demeaning or to tear down a colleague. The respect we are given as physicians comes with a responsibility to build people up, not put them down. This applies to colleagues as much as it does to patients. And if they are made to feel valued and comfortable, the quiet people on your team may just speak up and help you all with the task at hand. This is especially true of nurses, medical assistants, and patient care technicians, who are often the most reluctant to contribute.

Over time, the emotionally intelligent phrase *Is everything OK?* has also helped me focus other respected colleagues on their unproductive behaviors. Add *Is everything OK?* to your repertoire when confronted with colleagues who lack social grace, and be ready to accept the question's implicit hint when you're behaving out of character. *Is everything OK?* is a great way to bring attention to a behavior or situation that is not OK.

Reputation Is Built under Pressure

Drs. Mason and Brown were two surgery residents I met during neurosurgery rotations as a fourth-year medical student. Even though these men were only two or three years older than me, they seemed like demigods, the coolest people

I had ever met. I was about to become one of them, and I looked up to them with amazement.

Both were likable people who had done very well in medical school. Under calm circumstances, both were competent clinicians. I could see that their patients liked them. However, when circumstances turned stressful, they became different people—each in his own unique way.

Under pressure, Dr. Mason became arrogant. He micromanaged and belittled everyone around him. "You should know how to do this," he chided the intern. "It's fine, I'll do it myself," he snapped at the nurse. "I'm surrounded by amateurs," he muttered under his breath. I remember feeling sorry for those who had to endure his prickly nature. Within two weeks, Dr. Mason had alienated all his coworkers on every new rotation. Everyone dreaded working with him. No one relied on him or helped him. He was known for behaving badly during the worst moments—the stressful times when a patient's outcome was on the line.

Dr. Mason embodied Jekyll and Hyde characteristics, a behavioral pattern he probably learned from his mentors, as many of us do during training. Outside the operating room, he was jovial and under control, but under stress he turned nasty and mirrored Dr. Franklin's behavior. He sought admiration and respect, but somewhere in his training, he had adopted unprofessional coping mechanisms. As a rotating neurosurgery student, I observed his incongruent, odd behavior, and my respect turned to avoidance. On that rotation, I quietly lived and learned what *not* to do.

Dr. Brown also lost his nerve under pressure, but instead of exhibiting superiority, he panicked. He became an excitable Chicken Little, always afraid the sky was falling. There was a time he literally screamed "Help me!" in the middle of a code for cardiac arrest; the nurses just stood there, confused. When the pressure was on, he forgot all his checklists and struggled to do anything—he just froze. Not surprisingly, his colleagues did not consider him reliable. He didn't inspire confidence or trust.

Both surgeons had serious issues controlling their emotions. They didn't know how to cope. They were high-performing physicians who gave the best of themselves, except when circumstances didn't align with their expectations; then, their poor coping skills diminished their performance and therefore their reputations.

If you find yourself struggling with the same weakness, it's important to recognize that it's not the best version of yourself. The emotionally intelligent physician has the self-awareness to own that behavior and work to overcome it.

Don't feel guilty—chances are, you picked it up somewhere in training, watching people you admired. We all adopt behaviors such as that, gradually incorporating them into our identity. But sometimes they are poor representations of our full selves.

Everyone has moments of fear or indecision in crisis—you are human, after all. What you *do* in those moments determines your reputation. Are you someone who can be counted upon, the rock on whom others can depend? Or are you the problem in a crisis? Be mindful of your behaviors. The emotionally intelligent physician understands that managing chaos doesn't mean you act chaotically.

There will be situations in which you will feel uncertain of exactly what to do. The emotionally intelligent physician looks to the most experienced person in the room, whether

The real world is not about knowing the answer, but rather adapting to find and improve upon the answer.

that person is a nurse, a respiratory therapist, or another doctor, and asks them, "How can I help?" and then dons their gloves. "How can I help?" and the action of putting on the gloves demonstrate that you are looking to be part of the solution. Take the pressure off yourself through these actions by showing you are part of a team.

How about a situation in street clothes? I want you to take a quick deep breath and remember this acronym that I learned in my previous lives as an EMT first responder and a nursing assistant: ABC. No matter how chaotic or confusing the environment feels, every situation comes down to ABC: airway, breathing, and circulation. Someone on the airplane passes out: ABC. Someone at the mall falls down and starts to have a seizure: ABC. You're on the night float at the hospital by yourself and there's a code blue: ABC.

Stay calm and remember ABC, and you will save the patient. And enhance your reputation.

Be Perfectly Excellent

As part of my neurosurgery training, I rotated through the rigorous RUSH University transplant service. During that intense rotation, a new transplant surgeon joined the illustrious group. His impressive reputation preceded him. Dr. Nguyen had all the credentials: an Ivy League education and a prestigious residency program. He was articulate, knew the literature, and was poised—except in the operating room. There, under pressure, he blurted out obscene words. He cursed himself, the anatomy, and every surgical instrument.

He raised his voice to a level that made everyone in the room uncomfortable. He obsessed over small details that caused him to second-guess his surgical decisions.

Over time, the dark circles under Dr. Nguyen's eyes became more apparent. His shirt was always halfway untucked and his hair became more and more disheveled. Clearly, he was unraveling under the stress.

Dr. Nguyen's hard work, consistency, and dedication had brought him to excellence, but his obsession with perfection was now hurting him. "I can't make a mistake. This is someone's family member I'm taking care of," he would say. He rehearsed his actions repeatedly in his head, trying to get everything just right.

Perfection is a mantra in medical school training because we are evaluated on a finished product. But in the real world, patients and clinical scenarios are not finished products; they are unpredictable works in progress. The real world is not about knowing the answer, but rather adapting to find and improve upon the answer. Perfectionism sabotages good physicians.

In my opinion, perfectionism should be our default when taking a test, making an incision, or getting a haircut. In all other tasks, especially in the ever-changing dynamics of managing patients, speaking with families, and managing relationships with colleagues, *excellence* is the measure by which the extraordinary doctor should be judged. Excellence is built from small habits, all compounding and leading to great outcomes. The danger comes when those behaviors crystallize and the physician holds to a specific pattern even in the face of changing circumstances.

Ultimately, Dr. Nguyen was crushed by the weight of his own expectations. In chasing the respect of everyone around him and the false god of perfection in an imperfect world, he self-sabotaged and self-destructed. In an environment that required adaptability, the medical staff soon became concerned about his obsessive habits. Dr. Nguyen ended up taking a leave of absence and considering a career change. He was one of the most promising surgeons of his cohort, but a victim of his misplaced perfectionism.

Perfectionism is not always embodied by self-criticism, by the way. Sometimes perfectionists turn their ire on others. Physicians cursed by perfectionism will blame anyone and everything but themselves, to the point that they lose capacity for self-reflection: "The patient had the problem. The patient's anatomy was complicated." Obviously, there will be times when the issue genuinely is the patient's anatomy, but in my experience, these instances are rare. Physicians who insist that nothing is ever their fault cannot learn. They become so fragile that they cannot respond appropriately to circumstances that are out of their control. (And believe me— sometimes circumstances really are out of your control.)

The extraordinary doctor knows when to be perfect and, more importantly, when to be excellent.

How to Be Better

There is more to excellence than what we were taught in medical school. Clinical skills matter, but they are never enough. Extraordinary care requires emotional intelligence, having patience with people, and learning to think of the big picture. Patients and family members are overwhelmed because their future is in doubt. They crave trust. The superlative physician earns it when they address both the cognitive and emotional parts of the issue. Here are a few pearls on how to obtain trust.

- Addressing the physiological scenario is automatic, but trust is established by recognizing and acknowledging the psychological concern with a validation statement—for example, "I know this is difficult." Be able to also communicate the unknown element of the situation.

- In those emergent dire moments, the emotional part of a patient's or family member's brain takes precedence over the cognitive part, but the communication of the important risks, benefits, complications, and possible outcomes are all directed to the cognitive part of their brain. To obtain trust, we must also access their emotions. This is done through our calmness, cadence, and delivery while talking with them, not necessarily by providing the facts.

- Trust is defined by how you behave in stressful situations, not just by how you accomplish the clinical algorithm.

- There will be situations in which you will not know the next step. Keep your pride and display trust with humble and mature statements such as "Would you mind?" and "I don't know, but I'll find out."

In our profession, perfectionism is unavoidable and works well on concrete and finished products such as tests. However, patients, family members, and life-threatening situations are fluid and dynamic. Trust requires adaptability, and you will excel by striving for excellence. In the real world, perfectionism is self-sabotage. Knowing yourself becomes essential in our profession, where the rigid standards of perfectionism clash with the unpredictable realities of patient care and life-threatening situations.

4

Knowing Yourself Is a Competitive Advantage

———

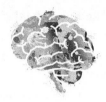

"I'VE BEEN SUED." Three words that strike fear into every physician's heart.

On a late Monday evening in 2019, I was driving home from work. The sun was setting on the Dallas skyline. Traffic was merciless, so to find my happy place, I chose the latest podcast on meditation. My phone chimed. It was Dr. Scott, a local surgeon I knew well.

"I want to run something by you," the text message read.

"Sure, I'll call you when I'm home," I responded.

I finally arrived home, hung out with my family, and called Dr. Scott when the kids went to bed.

After he answered, he said those three words that get every doctor's attention: "I've been sued."

"What happened?" I asked, baffled.

Dr. Scott and I had known each other for years. He was an excellent physician, pleasant to work with, even-keeled, and a valuable asset to his group. He gave articulate and easy-to-follow instructions and got along with everyone. With all these attributes, he had created a successful surgical practice. Dr. Scott was the full package.

I listened closely and kept silent for most of the conversation. By the speed and tempo of his speech, I could tell he was anxious. When he ended his deluge of details, he paused, took a breath, and said, "The lawyers have summoned me for a deposition. And I was hoping I could review the case with you."

"You got it," I said.

I was glad Dr. Scott had called me. My wife is a principal partner specializing in litigation for one of the largest global law firms. So I knew about litigation by osmosis. At this stage of my career, I was well acquainted with medical expert reviews. I had experience reading and drafting expert reports, participating in depositions, and offering testimony as a neurosurgery expert during trials. Additionally, I had served on physician behavior and discipline boards at both state and national levels.

I reviewed the events of Dr. Scott's case. He had been consulted to operate on a woman who was still suffering tremendous pain despite a prior spine operation by another surgeon. Upon review, I found no issues with Dr. Scott's surgical technique. His summary of the case was impeccable and articulate. The outcome was difficult—the woman's pain had not abated much—but it was a high-risk case. Medically speaking, the preoperative, intraoperative, and postoperative care were all excellent. At face value, the case was within what I considered to be the standard of care. So, why was he being sued?

As I continued to read the transcripts from his patient's deposition, I began to understand the trigger.

The patient said, "I never saw the doctor after the surgery. When I requested to see him instead of the nurse, the doctor seemed irritable." She continued, "The doctor told me, 'I took on the case when no one else would touch it. Your outcome isn't because of me.'"

This was his undoing. Dr. Scott was not being sued due to surgical errors; his technique was flawless. Instead, it was his dismissive demeanor that had led to legal action. He refused to acknowledge his role in the complication and, to compound matters, shifted *blame on to the patient*. The patient felt neglected and abandoned, making the lawsuit almost inevitable. If I were the patient, I'd be upset too.

In my view, there are two types of surgeons who claim they never encounter complications: those with limited experience and those who deceive themselves. Given Dr. Scott's considerable expertise, he fell into the latter category. He had been deceiving himself. Unfortunately, his lack of self-awareness prevented him from addressing the issue, exacerbating an already challenging situation.

The case eventually settled for a large amount, but the incident will haunt Dr. Scott for the rest of his career.

There are several key lessons that doctors can learn from Dr. Scott's experience:

1 Always make yourself reasonably available and maintain communication with your patient, especially when there is an unexpected outcome.

2 Be mindful of your demeanor and how it impacts patients and their families.

3 Do not deceive yourself; complications are a reality for every seasoned physician.

Why Knowing Yourself Matters

The outcome for Dr. Scott's patient proved challenging for both parties. As physicians, you will encounter unexpected outcomes. The mark of an extraordinary doctor is not how well you manage patients when outcomes are favorable; it is *how you manage them when outcomes are not favorable.*

Because of Dr. Scott's lack of self-awareness, how he treated his patient exacerbated her suffering. He was oblivious to his role in precipitating the lawsuit. Reflecting on our initial phone conversation, I realized he wasn't aware of this shortcoming at all. He never indicated responsibility; as far as Dr. Scott was concerned, the poor outcome was due to bad luck, and the patient's fault. While there might have been some truth to his perspective, his lack of empathy worsened an already difficult situation.

Physicians who ignore the importance of self-awareness will find themselves in trouble. We all make mistakes, but self-awareness allows us to acknowledge and rectify them, rather than deflecting blame elsewhere.

Understanding ourselves entails acknowledging the gaps in our knowledge and skills, confronting our failures, and recognizing how we are perceived by others. Think of it as performance optimization. It's the difference between experience and wisdom; it mitigates our weaknesses and prevents self-sabotage. Self-awareness will keep us from repeating the same mistakes.

The mark of an extraordinary doctor is how you manage patients when outcomes are not favorable.

Another way to think of it is as liability insurance—protection from ourselves.

The Competitive Advantage

A few years ago, two of my colleagues, Drs. Davidson and Raj, applied for the same leadership position of chief medical officer. This position meant managing hundreds of physicians and support staff, and facing high-pressure situations every day.

Dr. Davidson was the more tenured physician and actively engaged in hospital politics. He served on internal hospital committees, provided excellent patient care, and was fiscally astute. On paper, he was an impressive candidate. Unfortunately, his attitude sabotaged his advancement.

In the operating room, he assumed the role of authority, believing himself to be in charge. He directed the supporting medical staff to fall in line. The only problem was that his "my way or the highway" approach didn't sit well outside the confines of the operating room. At times, he was abrasive and overly assertive, even in non-emergency scenarios. While he achieved his objectives, his behavior caused friction among those around him.

Dr. Raj, too, was an excellent surgeon with a commanding presence in the operating room. He also served on hospital committees but maintained a lower profile in hospital politics. Like everyone else, Dr. Raj had his flaws, but what distinguished him was his ability to manage those imperfections.

Dr. Raj's nature was inherently reserved. But here's the thing: he knew when to hold back and when to step up. He actively sought feedback and adjusted accordingly, which gave him a significant advantage. On multiple occasions, Dr. Raj absorbed insights from operating room staff members or fellow surgeons. He praised nurses who identified mistakes by simply telling them "Thanks for catching that" and adjusting his and the team's approach accordingly.

Over time, Dr. Raj not only honed his technical prowess but also increased his influence—his people skills. His team deeply trusted him and would move mountains for him.

Both physicians were well suited to assume the chief medical officer role. Both were highly accomplished and well respected. But despite Dr. Raj being less seasoned, the hiring committee didn't hesitate to recognize his talents. He was promoted because of his openness to take in others' opinions and to adapt. The committee felt far more comfortable having someone in a position of authority who listened to the team and could adjust to changing circumstances than one who simply had more experience. They felt Dr. Raj's temperament and receptiveness would place the health system in safe hands.

By understanding his strengths and weaknesses, Dr. Raj had a competitive edge. He stood out because he listened and adapted. He didn't just push his own agenda right away. He prioritized understanding others' viewpoints. His self-awareness led to a significant advancement in his career.

Here's the unspoken truth: opportunities are always available for physicians who are balanced and self-aware. For the decision-makers, these individuals become their safest investment. Showcase these qualities and establish yourself as dependable. This will get you an invitation to a seat at the table.

"I'm sorry. We tried for hours, but we couldn't save her."

Dr. Kristoff was a senior emergency medicine resident at the university hospital in Louisville, Kentucky. She was speaking to a family in the trauma bay after a tragic accident. I could hear that her tone was low and heartfelt.

"She lost too much blood in transit."

The patient's mother started crying. The father stood up and stared at Dr. Kristoff for a long moment.

"I'm sorry," Dr. Kristoff repeated. "There was nothing any of us could do."

As though a switch were flipped, the husband's eyebrows angled in anger. His jaws became tense and he raised his voice sternly: "What are you talking about? You fix her now!" Then with an authoritative bellow, he repeated, "Now!" He stared wild-eyed at Dr. Kristoff.

His booming voice startled my colleagues and me. I stood there frozen, staring down at the concrete floor in embarrassment. I was anxious for Dr. Kristoff and a little frightened of this wild man. Fresh into my medical school rotations, I hadn't been taught anything to prepare me for such an intense moment.

Dr. Kristoff later told me that she had wanted to respond to the father but was aware it would likely escalate the situation. So instead, she stood still and said nothing. Nothing. She listened, doing her best to appear kind, nodding her head when he said something true, agreeing with him out loud when he said it was not fair. She didn't verbally retaliate when he threatened her. She did not walk away. She stood there, leaning into the moment, a silent witness to the man's raw anger.

The episode was tense and overwhelming. As security walked in the door, the father covered his face with his hands and started sobbing uncontrollably.

Dr. Kristoff's self-awareness that day allowed her to not take the incident personally. She recognized and, more importantly, controlled her emotions. She didn't let her or the man's emotions, or the hostile environment, control her. She choose to stay and to decide when she would walk away. Her outward, authoritative calm blunted the man's anger.

That day, Dr. Kristoff earned a legendary reputation with her colleagues. She had the self-awareness to monitor her own reactions and, as a result, shape her reputation.

Later that year, I met someone who lacked that self-knowledge: Dr. Julian. She was a new cardiology fellow who was consulted for cardiac clearance for a surgical patient. She arrived one morning to find that the short-staffed nursing team didn't have the patient ready for her evaluation. Dr. Julian glared at the nurse, slammed the chart on the desk, and left in a huff. In five minutes, when the patient *was* ready, the nursing team couldn't find her, and the surgery schedule fell even further behind.

Dr. Julian's tantrum affected her reputation. When the nurse gently broached the topic later that week, Dr. Julian became defensive, blaming her behavior on nursing incompetence. She finished her rant by saying that this happened every time she was consulted. Over time, she managed to keep her job, but she paid a high price by losing the respect of her support staff and colleagues.

Opportunities are
always available
for physicians who
are balanced
and self-aware.

Recognize Conflict *before* It Happens

Dr. Kristoff knew herself well enough to have a firm grasp on her emotions. Dr. Julian did not.

Self-awareness allows you to recognize a potential conflict a few milliseconds before it occurs. In that brief moment before the verbal joust, you are likely to feel a flash of emotions, including images of potential consequences. Being able to foresee this *before* it happens will put you in the driver's seat to make better decisions.

You will also self-regulate your emotional states up or down in response to the environment. You can adjust to switch from verbal to nonverbal communication, such as silence and nodding your head, as Dr. Kristoff exhibited, to support the outcomes you desire. Self-awareness becomes an internal corrective mechanism, if you listen.

In the previous chapter, I described how as a young physician, I made a fool of myself by refusing to admit I didn't know how to properly insert an NG tube. Ignorance wasn't the issue there; the issue was my lack of self-awareness. I refused to admit to myself what I didn't know, and therefore I chose not to ask for help. My pride, and my shoes, took the resulting punishment. That day, I papered over my lack of experience to maintain my ego.

Similarly, when questioned about her availability, to maintain her own ego, Dr. Julian insulted the nurse. If ego trips us up, it becomes dangerous.

To be clear, ego itself is not the problem. Our profession requires a certain level of healthy ego and pride. We need to display confidence in the face of uncertainty and to be psychologically resilient in the face of challenge. That takes a strong ego. However, the difference between a strong, positive ego and a strong, negative, fragile ego is self-awareness. How you present yourself—whether it's with genuine confidence or its opposite, imposter syndrome—hinges on self-awareness. Others can sense these nuances through your demeanor.

Sooner or later, every physician will face a serious test. How will you behave when challenged? Will you rise to the occasion with confidence, or will you crumble? Fortunately, if you come to that test as well prepared as you did for your MCATS, armed with self-awareness and a healthy ego, you will make better choices.

Even as practicing physicians, we will continue to encounter significant tests, but those challenges appear in another form. Being prepared by knowing yourself will navigate you through seven common scenarios that frequently arise in medical practice. We'll look at those next.

5

Seven Scenarios You Need to Prepare For

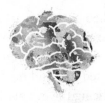

"Excuse me, passengers, the captain is requesting a doctor to assist with an emergency. Please press the call light so the attendant can find you."

Ding, Ding, Ding

The quiet dark cabin allowed me to hear the chorus of call light volunteers. *Situation controlled*, I thought, pulling the blanket over my head.

Little did I know that my loving and proactive wife had pushed my call light and even flagged down the attendant.

"He can help." I felt her arm pointing over me.

I had spent a few years practicing in the real world, saving up some money along the way. It was my first time in first class, a gift for our wedding anniversary. We were headed to a safari in South Africa. I had donned every first-class amenity offered. Why not?

The attendant pulled back the curtain and motioned for me to follow down the aisle. It took a moment for my dilated pupils to adjust from the darkness of my seat. As I emerged, searing sunlight greeted me, and my fellow travelers fixed their eyes on me, noticing the eye mask draped around the neck of my airline pajamas. I froze in the awkward moment. The flight attendant tugged at my sleeve, and we swiftly moved to the passenger. The attendant handed me a container that resembled a fishing tackle box: needles, syringes, and a boatload of medications I hadn't seen in years. There was a nice little instruction manual written in a foreign language.

I swallowed hard, sifted through the cobwebs in my brain, and heard the EMT within echo, "When was the last time you started an IV, brother? ABC, ABC, ABC."

The passenger made it through the flight. The flight attendant crew rewarded me with a self-selected complimentary bottle of Johnnie Walker Blue. It was polished off before we made it to our destination.

Every plane comes with instructions on how to buckle your seatbelt, plus a laminated placard on how to inflate a raft for an emergency water landing. There's even an indecipherable little manual for the emergency tackle box.

But an essential guide on how to handle tricky scenarios for lifesaving doctors in the real world? We have none.

Until now. Here are seven common scenarios you will likely face in your practice. I still face some of these situations after my many years in practice. And to be honest, I don't always excel in them the first time, despite considering myself an experienced and self-aware physician.

As you read each scenario, take some time to think about your personality. What will be your most likely natural tendency in that circumstance? What, if anything, should you do instead?

Knowing what you should do in advance doesn't mean you will automatically execute as hoped, but it sure will keep you one step ahead of trouble.

Scenario 1: The Offending Question

It was Labor Day weekend, and I was called to the emergency room to evaluate an eighteen-year-old college student who had suffered a severe open skull fracture in a Jet Ski accident. By the time I saw him, it was clear he needed immediate brain surgery.

People feel comforted when their surgeon walks into the room and is weathered, with gray hair, and at least appears as if he has been doing this longer than they have been alive. That wasn't me. I was near the beginning of my career. While new practicing physicians often look young, for some reason I appeared even younger than most. I was in my early thirties, but my gangly build and boyish face made me look more like a teenager.

The family politely listened as I explained the concerning issue with the brain, the risks of the surgery, and that we had to operate immediately.

Then the mother asked me in a hesitating voice, "You have... you have done this before?"

I was offended. She had no right to question my skill set after my near-decade of training. I had earned the right to be there and was trained to have excellent knowledge and surgical skills. I resented the implication.

Remember
the Golden Rule:
treat others as
you would like
others to treat you.

There were two ways I could handle this question. Door One: My unchecked amygdala response could have thrown down a searing "Listen, I've got this handled. I wouldn't be here if I didn't know what I was doing." But at this point in my career, I knew success in moving her son forward to surgery was not behind that door. She would shut down, possibly call for another opinion, or slow down the decision in some other way. She would seek to alleviate the real and understandable anxiety we all felt—and her son did not have that kind of time. His life was actually on the line.

So instead, at some cost to my ego, I chose Door Two: Let the offense go. I acknowledged the mother's feelings the best way I knew how at that time. I said, "Ma'am, I understand this is a tough situation for everyone. And yes, this is a high-risk procedure. But this is the world I live in. This is what I've been trained to do."

I finished our dialogue calmly, answering all her questions. I assured her that our team was comfortable with the operation and that we would do everything we could to make sure her son did well. The mother calmed down, and I could see she would at least accept the idea of trusting me.

Looking back, I now understand that her question was not a judgment of my competence. It simply reflected her emotional angst in a difficult situation and her fear of the unknown. Her son's life was hanging in the balance, and the man who was about to operate on him barely appeared to be a man, let alone a seasoned surgeon.

The right answer, as hard as it can be, is not to take these feelings personally. Instead, address the underlying emotional issue at play.

What I learned from this experience was the importance of connecting before consulting. I connected with the mother by prioritizing her emotions and acknowledging the difficult situation she was in before discussing the medical details. When people feel heard, they are more likely to take in what you need to convey.

Connect before consulting: address the emotion in the room.

Scenario 2: Dr. Google

Many patients will have done their research before they come to visit you for their clinic appointment. Their resources will be a plethora of incomplete information, typically bits and pieces from family and friends or even local organizations, such as work or church.

My favorite is "Dr. Google." I have found that more than offering solutions, Dr. Google leaves patients asking more questions. Truthfully, I, too, have investigated Dr. Google for the conditions I treat. And the information available in layman's terms is confusing even for me. A few clicks and the word "cancer" inevitably appears. Patients have come to my clinic certain that their diagnosis is cancer or maybe some rare pig parasite from Brazil, when in fact it is something else.

I have learned to become more understanding and adaptable with my responses in these common scenarios. Some of the information makes sense to me, and some… well… has left me questioning their resources. Early in my career, I reacted to off-the-beaten-path information with a slightly dismissive undertone. In one situation, I interrupted a patient who presented me with a folder of research documents. I flipped through the pages in the folder and curtly responded, "No, that's a bunch of BS. They don't know what they're talking about." The patient's response was almost entirely nonverbal. I could see that they felt deflated. I sounded full of myself.

My impatience prevented me from delivering excellent patient care on that day, and I regretted being dismissive. My response now is more supportive, or at least neutral. Common responses I use today include:

- "Wow. That's interesting."
- "I like that."
- "Great job on doing the homework."

For these patients, I have found success in commending their efforts instead of criticizing their information. Acknowledging patients for taking ownership of their medical condition is a great way to connect before explaining the reality of the situation. Which rarely involves a pig parasite from Brazil.

Scenario 3: "But the Other Doctor Said..."

Like Mrs. Dionne, a sixty-four-year-old active woman with back and leg pain, patients may seek you for a second opinion. Mrs. Dionne was a surgical candidate who came to me to verify that she indeed needed surgery.

During my evaluation, she interrupted, saying, "But the other surgeon said... Why did they say this?"

I remember, first, not enjoying being interrupted and, second, feeling uninterested in comparing my thoughts with another surgeon.

In my early years, my earnest desire to stretch the extra mile to help the patient understand "the other opinion" led to assumptions that were unfortunately incomplete. I have learned to instead focus directly on the scenario in front of me. Instead of meandering down the unknown road of another physician's opinion, I now respond with "Thank you for sharing that with me. But I can't speak to the other physician's thoughts. Based on my evaluation of you, I recommend..." This approach kindly notifies the patient that I am not willing to cross the line of professionalism.

Speculating on another physician's opinion without understanding the full context of the physician-patient conversation breaches an unspoken code of conduct of our profession. There are subtle nuances with each patient interaction that direct a physician's opinion. I wouldn't want another physician opining on my diagnosis and treatment plan without having a full understanding of what I observed and evaluated. Remember the Golden Rule: treat others as you would like others to treat you.

Scenario 4: "I'm Worse Off"

It's inevitable. Sometimes your tireless efforts will have unexpected outcomes. People who should get better just do not. They tell you they are "worse off." That's reality.

There have been moments when I felt defeated after doing everything I could for my patient. It could have been a combination of the disease process itself, their physically deconditioned status, and their psychological state that prevented the desired outcome. I have been surprised to learn that sometimes a secondary influence prevents a good outcome. Experience has taught me that there are obvious and not-so-obvious influences that can affect patient results.

I take time and effort to ensure that each patient has the best outcome possible. My professional identity is tied to that outcome, so I will sacrifice whatever it takes to get it right. Patients trust me, and I take that trust seriously.

That doesn't mean I don't also strive to understand moments of personal failure after operating on a patient. Mr. Smith came to the clinic and complained of low back and bilateral leg pain. He had failed nonoperative treatment for months and was quite miserable. The MRI of his lumbar spine demonstrated severe stenosis. I diagnosed Mr. Smith with lumbar stenosis causing neurogenic claudication and recommended lumbar surgery. The surgery was accomplished as planned, and I was satisfied with the results. I spoke with the family afterward and assured them that I expected him to feel better.

For the two-week follow-up appointment, I was eager to see Mr. Smith and his family. I walked into the room in an upbeat fashion and asked, "Well, how are things?"

Mr. Smith responded in an accusatory and disappointed tone. "I am worse off than before surgery. I am just beside myself that I had the surgery."

Now, I was not expecting that response, and truthfully, his comment was hurtful. I'm not in the business of making patients worse. Did they not understand the intense emotional energy it took for me to try to help him? His surgery was no walk in the park. I worked hard to take care of him.

Internally, I was irritated. I wanted to look him in the eye and respond, "You are ungrateful." And then tersely give him reasons why he should be grateful. Instead of feeling proud of how I took care of him, I felt as if I had done something malicious.

At that moment, I had a choice. I could respond at the same level of his anger—and believe me, I wanted to. However, I was the authority in the room, and if I belittled him in return, I would do so from a perceived position of power. Nothing good would have come from that. Perhaps I could have been dismissive and told him that the outcome was his problem and blamed his body. (Sound familiar?) That would've been a great countermove. I'd feel better, but he'd leave feeling much worse. A no-win situation there as well.

Instead, I chose to validate his feelings and then express *my* feelings. Validating someone is saying, explicitly or implicitly, that their feelings and experience are heard. It is possible to validate someone's feelings and still disagree with their conclusions or actions. In this case, I said, "I understand you are frustrated. I am just as disappointed as you are." I took him through everything I had accomplished, driven by a sincere desire to help. The walk-through helped him better understand but did not satisfy his expectations. At least it was progress—and more importantly, I avoided making a bad situation worse.

Ultimately, Mr. Smith improved and the whole exchange was water under the bridge. Sometimes you just need to buy time without further complicating the issue at hand.

Self-awareness
gives you the
ability to mitigate
your mistakes.

Scenario 5: It's the Right Thing to Do

I was a fourth-year medical school student rotating in the honors surgery program at the University of Louisville. The second-year surgery resident manning the ICU all night looked weary. He had been putting out a lot of patient fires.

At 6 a.m., the whole general surgery division gathered at the door of the first ICU patient. Today we were having the famous "Polk Rounds," led by the notable chairman of surgery, Dr. Hiram Polk. The resident stood at attention with confidence and began his presentation of ICU Patient No. 1. A dialogue ensued between the resident and the pharmacist about whether the patient should be on antibiotics. Ultimately, the resident ended the conversation with "It's the right thing to do." I remember the dismayed look on the pharmacist's face.

By saying it was the right thing to do, the resident had unintentionally implied that the pharmacist did not want to do the right thing. Be mindful of this phrase. If you do feel your idea or action is in the best interest of the patient, say, "In my experience, I have seen..." or "This is what has worked for me in the past." By stating your idea from an unquestionable experience, you will be effectively delivering your message without stepping on anyone else's toes.

Scenario 6: Shooting the Messenger

It was 6:56 a.m., just four minutes from the end of my on-call shift, and my phone buzzed *again*. I was exhausted, irritable, hungry; I had operated all night and was counting the minutes until the end of my call shift. But the dawn brought on a new day, and a normal full day's work lay ahead of me.

"Dr. Patel, I have a consult for you," the tired resident on the other end of the line politely stated.

"What time did the patient come in?" I demanded. "How long have they been here? Why are you calling me now? This is a bad consult."

I found myself unloading a barrage of verbal bullets at this young resident physician with all my frustrations from a tough night.

The resident took a moment to collect herself and then—despite an emotionally difficult situation—responded with poise. "Dr. Patel, thank you for taking the call. What is the best way to let you know about a consult in the future?"

Boom. I was embarrassed and felt put in my place. I had acted like a child, and she had responded like an adult. I apologized to her, and we did the consult.

There will be times in your career when the demands exceed what you believe you can offer. You will be tired. You will be beaten up. And someone will need you at what seems to be the worst time. It's in these moments that you may sense a profound isolation, as if your struggles go unnoticed and unacknowledged.

In that whirlwind of emotions, you may feel consumed with anger and irritation. How you choose to respond in that moment matters.

The resident turned a negative situation into a learning experience. Retaliating would have been far less productive than professionally and gently making me aware of my short-comings, as she did.

A week later, the same resident happened to call again just minutes before my call shift was over. Fatigue, irritability, and dwindling patience dominated my persona. This time, however, I managed the situation differently. I recalled a new acronym I had recently learned: HALT. It served as a reminder to check for hunger, anger, loneliness, and tiredness—the four pillars of emotional vulnerability. It was a mental cue that prompted communication between my frontal lobes and amygdala, helping me avert any potential self-destructive reactions. And I am proud to say that this time, I modified my response: I took the information calmly and thanked her warmly.

The need for self-awareness remains constant. The best you can do is become comfortable with this reality. We all make mistakes. Self-awareness gives you the ability to mitigate your mistakes—in this scenario, it was to not beat up the same resident twice.

Scenario 7: The Quality Review

Sooner or later, every physician providing patient care in a hospital will encounter a case subject to quality review. My cases have been reviewed by a quality committee, and now I participate in reviewing cases as a member of the quality committee.

A seventeen-year-old male presented to the emergency room with quadriplegia: he was unable to move his arms and legs. He had been pulled out of a shallow pool by friends after diving in headfirst and breaking his neck. We rushed him to the operating room and operated all night, trying tirelessly to save his spinal cord function. Unfortunately, he remained unable to move his arms and legs.

It was a complex case destined for a poor outcome despite our heroic efforts. When I received notification that it was under a quality review, I couldn't help but feel irritated. The review process felt personal. The physicians reviewing the case were my peers, and I resented feeling judged by them. I was embarrassed and defensive.

What I have learned time and time again is that the quality review is not all about the facts. Yes, the facts are important and are scrutinized long before you enter the room. But here's the secret. The peer review is more about how you respond to the questions. Your peers will formulate an impression—and therefore an assessment—by how you handle yourself.

After the review was over, I learned that the case was about what could have been done better—a process improvement. Great organizations are constantly looking for ways to improve. No one was blaming me or the team for the poor outcome; the hospital just wanted to know if there were ways to handle such cases better in the future. But my ultimate takeaway happened when Dr. Simon, the chairman of the peer review committee, found me sitting at the physicians' lounge table sipping on my coffee in between surgical cases. He pulled out a chair from the table, sat down, and leaned over.

"Hey, Nimesh, we'd like for you to serve on the quality committee with us," Dr. Simon said. "I'm not gonna lie, it's a time commitment. But you're the kind of physician we need—conscientious and professional."

After ten years and a plethora of quality review cases, I can tell you this: physicians often take reviews personally because, understandably, we perceive our work to be a reflection of ourselves. That is the inherent nature of any accomplished individual. The key is to know how you tend to behave and to move past it.

Peer reviews are inevitable. Although they can feel like punitive measures, they are instead proactive ones to improve the quality of health care overall. Our conduct in response to these reviews shapes how we are perceived and treated in return.

Remember that little secret: a quality review is more about how you respond and behave than the actual facts of the case.

I challenge you to embark on focused self-exploration specifically for physicians. This next chapter will require candid introspection of your personal ambition and professional identity. As you read it, I encourage you to embrace the transformative power of self-awareness, which will open a path toward authenticity and fulfillment in your medical practice.

6

Finding What Motivates You to Perform at Your Best

———

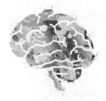

GREW UP in a small town in Kentucky, where my parents managed a motel. Our place was pretty basic, and our car had definitely seen better days. Meanwhile, a kid named Brian sported those Ralph Lauren polo shirts everyone wanted, and Darrin rocked brand-new Guess jeans. Me? My folks couldn't fathom splurging on such pricey cool attire. But Brian, being a generous guy, offered up his old polo shirts.

My upbringing and background shaped my views on resilience, resourcefulness, and material wealth. Becoming a neurosurgeon wasn't some grand plan. I started off medical school without a clue about neurosurgery or what a neurosurgeon even did. Turned out, I was all about surgery. Identifying strategies and fixing problems using my hands to sort things out probably comes from my days fixing bike chains and brakes.

In my last year of neurosurgery training, I received a job offer via email while sitting in the ICU at Lutheran General during my trauma rotation. I giggled. I had never even dreamed of making so much money, and for something I enjoyed doing. It felt unreal—dreams of a big house, my own polo shirts... and forget the jeans! But I vividly remember having mixed feelings of excitement, a touch of shame, and determination to earn some respect.

Fast-forward twenty years, and I now realize how some old psychological wounds can trap us in unexpected ways. The allure of the nice salary, luxurious possessions, and comfortable lifestyle that come with the profession may have helped heal some lingering feelings of inadequacy. And there is no shame in wanting material comfort, to be sure. But here's the deal: once you attain what you've always desired materially, your definition of what constitutes success may transform. It can help, from the start, to understand the immaterial markers that distinguish this profession as well.

Every human wants authority, respect, and relevance in their own lives. The moment we become doctors, people intrinsically grant us those qualities. The emotionally intelligent, extraordinary doctor comes to understand that they have a responsibility to live up to the special status conferred on them, to the best of their ability.

To achieve this, you may need to dive deeper to understand what motivated you to pursue a career in medicine in the first place, including the less than altruistic impulses, so you don't succumb to them.

On my journey, I've seen the darker side of motivations, the pressures and doubts and the tangled road, which has slowly transformed into a more genuine path.

Why Did You Become a Doctor?

When you find yourself with a free moment, ask yourself, "Why did I choose to be a doctor?"

There's no wrong answer, just the truth. And knowing the truth will help you know yourself and your inner motivations better.

When I asked myself this question, I first looked to my medical school application. What I wrote there was noble and idealistic, but I didn't see those exact ideals play out in the years that immediately followed. I've since learned that people and life can be beautiful *and* cruel. Both things can be true and coexist at the same time.

If you resonate with my experience, perhaps you pursued a career in medicine as a way out, or for the status and perks. Maybe you craved the prestige, being admired and relevant, or the economic security. Most of us are driven by a combination of those factors. Be honest with yourself. None of these motivations are good or bad, but their allure can be seductive. The emotionally intelligent physician examines their motivations with eyes wide open. Being mindful of the driving forces behind your actions will make you more vigilant against the pitfalls that come along with them (which we'll talk about below).

Maybe you chose this profession because it was considered the norm. Have you ever asked yourself why? Thinking through the following highly personal questions helped me gain better understanding.

- **Am I motivated by the money?** How important was financial security? I wanted to make a good living. While I might have outwardly downplayed its importance, deep down, I yearned for the financial stability I never had in my youth.

- **Am I intrigued by the science?** Did I have the spirit of an architect or engineer? Some physicians view medicine as an enjoyable puzzle solved with intricate algorithms. I could help people by applying science to real-life situations. This could fulfill my passion for tinkering.

- **Am I here out of a sense of legacy?** Was there someone important in my life who was a physician? Perhaps I saw how much respect they received for it or the noble air they carried. I wanted to emulate them.

- **Am I here because I was inspired?** Did I see tragedy up close? Did disease take a loved one from me and I felt a calling into health care? Am I trying to answer the question of how to make a difference in this world?

I was driven by a number of these dynamics. The internal dialogue helped me discern my genuine motivations. On the cloudy days, the self-reflective answers kept me resilient, and on the bright days, they helped me stay humble and grateful.

I started to track my motivations by simply noticing behavior and thoughts as they happened. What do you notice? What patterns do you see? What tendencies do you have in certain circumstances? Get used to watching your thoughts and behaviors as they occur.

Once you develop familiarity, begin the following cognitive optimization and self-assessment practices.

The emotionally intelligent physician examines their motivations with eyes wide open.

The Pitfalls of Motivation

Delving into the potential pitfalls and drawbacks of the various driving forces can help you be cognizant of the downsides of your tendencies. Too much unrecognized motivation can lead you down a path you will regret. On the flip side, understanding your motivations can help you optimize your performance.

When we lose sight of the nobility inherent in our profession, it's tempting to let negativity seep into our lives. Remember, the true focus is not on us. Instead, we physicians are viewed as conduits between a higher purpose and those who are desperate, weak, and forgotten. I truly believe this unspoken public perception now, though I can't say I always understood it when I was younger.

While financial success is a valid aspiration, those motivated by money should be mindful of the ethical pitfalls. If we justify clinical decisions based on financial reward, we could too easily wake up one day realizing that we have done something we regret.

As "tinkerers," we tend to view everyone as a tinker toy. The risk is that we can become so fascinated with science that we ignore the human aspect. We need to keep in mind that we are treating patients and their families, all of whom have feelings and concerns. Half of healing is psychological. Remember, we are created as emotional creatures capable of logic, not logical creatures capable of emotion. Simply addressing the physical ailment reduces us to mere technicians.

The weight of legacy from generations can lead to a myopic focus on the self. We seek to imprint everything that is touched. Legacy seekers spend their days chasing self-validation and influence at the cost of the work that brought them to this point. We self-delude that image is enough, but that image will crumble if the work diminishes in its quality. Even the image will eventually fade.

Vengeance seekers or martyrs will incessantly fight injustice and disease but may inadvertently neglect self-care. Burnout becomes a looming risk as they confront the harsh reality that life is inherently unfair. They may obsess over helping others while ignoring their personal well-being and fulfillment.

Understanding yourself on a profound level reveals the hazards of unconscious motivation. You will anticipate the traps and be able to sidestep them. Recognizing these vulnerable tendencies will help address your weaknesses and evolve you into an extraordinary, emotionally intelligent physician.

Early in my career, I wish I had set clear definitions of personal and professional success. What does success mean in one year, five years, a decade? Is it about finances, a specific title, or mastering your schedule? Define it, pursue it, but remember: once you've achieved a goal, don't let it dictate your life by incessantly seeking more of the same. There are diminishing returns once you exceed a certain threshold.

Be Better Today Than Yesterday

What can you do to improve yourself and optimize your performance? There are a number of steps you can take. I outline the processes that worked for me below. You can adapt these to suit your personality or come up with additional rituals on your own.

Subtract Instead of Add

There's nothing more dreadful than coming off a wonderful call-free weekend only to have Monday morning punch me in the mouth. Emergency consults, a slew of unanswered emails, and of course my regularly scheduled morning program yet to be accomplished. In this situation, and many others, I have learned to improve my mindset by exercising self-awareness.

The process is easy. Instead of adding a mandatory behavior to an already full plate, such as striving to be positive, I now subtract a behavior—for example, *not* being negative.

My logic is that refraining from doing something is less cognitively demanding than doing something, and focusing on a specific item will aid my mindset. "I will eat healthy," for instance, is too broad, while the more specific "I will not eat sugar" is easier to achieve.

A simple change of perspective can make a significant difference.

Journal for Focus

I started journaling a few years ago solely to improve my self-performance. I was never a writer or reader, but I wanted to become a clear and concise communicator. As a hypothesis tester, I committed to journaling once a day for three weeks. Years later, I still journal regularly, and I give journals out to my friends and colleagues who are trying to connect with their best selves.

The act of writing, even today, allows me to access subconscious parts of my brain. I began by merely filling out journal prompts. Some days I had no motivation to write and simply wrote that sentiment. But I soon discovered that the pen took on a life of its own. Experiencing this subconscious flow was truly remarkable. Journaling opens up secret corridors that help me categorize complex situations into bite-sized ideas. The process connects me to my goals and allows me to recognize and manage unwanted behavior more easily. Best of all, by eliminating mental detritus as I write the words down, I free up my energy and focus.

My process is simple: I write, review, and write again. In the beginning, there were days when I didn't know what to write, but I kept my hand moving. I found things that I could never have foreseen. Stream of consciousness writing is straightforward, but you must do it regularly to see the biggest benefits.

The most powerful and revealing part of the process comes when you review what you write. If you put in the effort, you can realize things about yourself you did not even know existed. You will recognize behavioral patterns. Your motivation. Self-sabotaging behavior. This is the place where you will discover these keys to your psychology.

Practice Mindful Meditation

Earlier I mentioned Dr. Julian, the cardiology fellow who became rude with the nurses after being on call. There was also Dr. Kristoff in the emergency room, who stood there while an upset father berated her, and my story about the day I became perturbed at the resident after a night on call.

The difference between Dr. Julian, Dr. Kristoff, and me was not our emotions. If anything, Dr. Kristoff's inward emotions may have been stronger, as she was facing an angry family

Knowing yourself
will optimize your
performance and help
you get more
of what you want.

member and was concerned he might escalate to violence. All of us felt a threat, and all of us faced a potential fight-or-flight response mediated by the amygdala in our brains.

When we face a threat, even a low-level confrontation, *especially* when we are tired and hungry at the end of a demanding shift, our prefrontal cortex can loosen its control. In other words, the amygdala "hijacks" the brain. (The term "amygdala hijack" was first coined by Daniel Goleman in his 1995 book *Emotional Intelligence: Why It Can Matter More Than IQ*.) The fight-or-flight impulse drives our actions.

Let me back up for a moment to review brain science. If you recall, the amygdala is our evolutionary emotional hub. It processes emotion and memories associated with fears. It is designed to respond to threats. It cannot discern the difference between minor and major threats. When the amygdala hits a certain level of excitation, you "snap." Emotion takes over the brain, and you are thrown into a fight-or-flight state.

In contrast, the prefrontal cortex is the CEO of our brains. It is rational and considerate. It controls behavior and attention, and—when it is functioning normally—it can inhibit the raw impulses of the amygdala. But the prefrontal cortex is not perfect.

The difference between people who "snap" at low levels of threat (like Dr. Julian and me that day) and those who can remain calm even in the face of high levels of threat (like ER physician Dr. Kristoff, and Dr. Julian and me on a better day) is the difference in the inhibitory ability of the prefrontal cortex. The prefrontal cortex did more "heavy lifting" to stay in control of the amygdala in the second cases.

If you want to increase your prefrontal cortex's inhibitory ability to "lift," you will need to practice inhibition. Studies show that mindfulness meditation allows you to do exactly that. Over time, a mindfulness meditation habit creates a more even-keeled, more focused, less reactionary brain. The meditator's prefrontal cortex is more in control and less able to be pushed around by impulse and threats to the ego. Mindfulness meditation helps you know yourself.

Mindfulness is not difficult and can take several forms. The classic form is sitting, closing your eyes, and doing a breathing exercise for a few minutes while you empty your mind. I personally have found focus and clarity from writing, exercising, and long mindful walks.

Surprisingly, scientific studies have demonstrated that as little as two minutes can make a difference in the brain's wiring. Functional MRI studies have demonstrated neuroplastic changes in the physical brain. The brains of long-term meditators show that EEG waves move to more optimal frequencies.

I believe meditation allows conscious access to the processing power of the subconscious, since long-time meditators have more alpha and beta waves apparent in the EEG. These brain waves most commonly spike in the space between wakefulness and sleep; they are the markers of the subconscious mind. The effects of meditation can be proved by science.

Devoted meditators can access alpha and beta wave states deliberately. They are able to evoke more creativity and focus and to understand problems at a deeper, more intuitive level. This makes sense, since the subconscious mind is capable of filtering and understanding a much larger quantity of information than the conscious mind.

The extraordinary doctor can control their emotions through practices such as meditation.

Steady Your Nerves with Box Breathing

Snipers and Navy Seals use box breathing before they act in clutch situations. In high-risk scenarios, neurosurgeons also employ box breathing, to calm their hands before putting a clip on a brain aneurysm, for instance. Find a way to utilize this technique to calm yourself in a stressful situation.

Meta-analysis data suggests that box breathing actually changes the autonomic nervous system, specifically the parasympathetic response and specific brain waves on EEG readings—the brain waves that lead to more focus, reduced anxiety, and improved vigor.

Box breathing is most effective when you are already anxious, so again, knowing yourself is key to realizing when you need this intervention. You must be able to recognize the signs of your own emotional stress to address that stress with box breathing.

For example, before I step on stage for public speaking, my heart races and my voice tightens. In the past, I have recognized my nerves and completed a round of box breathing to calm them. These days, because I am aware of how many times this pattern has happened, I use the breathing technique prophylactically.

Box breathing is simple. Visualize a four-sided box. With your mind's eye, walk your eyes across the top of the box while inhaling for four seconds. Hold that breath while moving your eyes down the right side of the box for four seconds. Now exhale for four seconds while walking your eyes across the bottom of the box. Then with your lungs empty, let your eyes travel up the left side of the box. In this way, you will complete a circuit of the box: inhale 1-2-3-4, hold 1-2-3-4, exhale 1-2-3-4, hold 1-2-3-4. Repeat this circuit three times to gain the effect of this technique.

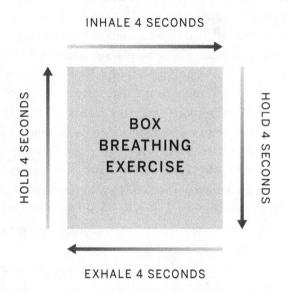

INHALE 4 SECONDS

HOLD 4 SECONDS

BOX BREATHING EXERCISE

HOLD 4 SECONDS

EXHALE 4 SECONDS

Dance with the Voice in Your Head

The voice in your head is likely your worst critic. Contrary to what the "hand waving" social media gurus out there say, changing that voice takes significant cognitive behavioral therapy, which is beyond the scope of this book. Instead of changing that voice, I want to tell you how to dance with it.

When I woke up to that gut punch of a phone call saying "Sorry, Nimesh, you didn't match," during my fourth year of medical school (see the book's introduction for this story), the voice in my head was cruel, and it can still resurface in hard times. *Am I an imposter even after all these years?* Back then, people would tell me, "Don't be so hard on yourself," as if I could stop the inner critic just by willing it. Obviously, I could not. But out of pure emotional survival, I learned to befriend it instead.

The truth is that the voice of my self-criticism has been there for my victories as well as my failures. It's not going away. Given our ongoing relationship, we could not continue to be at odds; we just had to change how we spoke to each other. And now we dance. I made a deal with that voice. My role was to step up to the plate whether I failed or not. In return, the voice was welcomed and appreciated, with a caveat: it could tell me how badly I had failed, but it also had to tell me how to get better.

We are always a work in progress. Remember that when you start to judge yourself too critically.

Ask What Others Think

Knowing yourself is not just about self-knowledge; it's also knowing how you are perceived by others. It's impossible to understand others' perceptions of you without asking them. I want you to ask them.

At the beginning of my foray into health care administration, I started to moderate meetings and present to various hospital boards. Both of these tasks were, to me, new skills with high stakes. I wanted to make a good impression and needed to understand how I presented myself. The only way to know was to ask, so after each meeting or presentation, I privately approached someone who was there for a postmortem.

"What did you think of the presentation?" I asked.

At times, I worried that instead of coming across as assertive and knowledgeable, I might be perceived as unsure and lacking in confidence. Sometimes the person confirmed my worry, and sometimes they gave me other feedback. Whether positive or negative, I listened to that feedback and acted on it, trying to improve my presentation skills over time.

I recommend that you use the same technique to get to know yourself better and optimize your performance. Postmortems are useful when you are developing new skills, and building a base understanding of your tendencies, strengths, and weaknesses from people you trust is also important. If you know your shortcomings, you will not keep running into the wall. We can't satisfy everyone and their opinions, but it's good to canvass what is out there.

Over time, I developed a personal advisory board. Doing this is simple, since people love to give their opinions. Recruit at least three reliable people, preferably trusted colleagues whom see you often. At least one should be a peer, as close to your age and role as possible. Having two peers is even better—they can provide fact-checks for each other. One person gives a hypothesis, and the other stress tests that hypothesis.

Combine any of these questions.

- How would you describe my demeanor?
- How do I come across when I am stressed and angry?
- How do I proceed when I do not know the answer?
- How do I come across when I am nervous?
- How do I behave when my authority has been challenged?

Asking a trusted person for this specific information requires humility. It means accepting whatever information you hear, good impressions or bad. The truth is always the right place to start the thinking process. It's like having a car inspected—it's a self-diagnosis intended to help you improve and be ready for the long road ahead.

Once you know your baseline, you will be in a better position to anticipate your tendencies, plan for them, and modify them as necessary.

The key is to choose people whose opinion you respect. You want to be motivated to act on what you learn rather than dismiss it.

Investing in Self-Knowledge Is Worth It

Knowing yourself is one of the most difficult skills for anyone to learn. But if you commit to it, you will have more control over who you become. This skill will give you a competitive advantage. Think of it as a psychological Swiss Army knife. It will separate the lemming from the leader, the commodity from the person in control, the mediocre from the extraordinary, fulfilled physician. Do you want to be the exception or the rule?

Knowing yourself will keep you out of trouble. We're in a high-stakes profession. Complications will happen, either directly because of you or associated with you. There are only two kinds of surgeons who don't have complications: liars and those who haven't done much. Again, the measure of a great physician is not the capacity to manage patients when they are doing well, but rather the capacity to manage them when they are not. Understand how you behave when things don't go your way.

Knowing yourself will optimize your performance and help you get more of what you want. Being self-aware means seeing the future a millisecond before it happens. If you are about to enter a confrontational conversation, understanding your body movement, speech, and interaction will help you predict a proactive behavior, not a reactionary behavior.

Knowing yourself will open your career for advancement opportunities. You will be seen as a role model inside and outside the hospital. The question will be whether or not you want to accept that role. If you do, the way you listen, react, and handle yourself will be on display. Those individuals who have poise will always be considered for a seat at the table.

In the next chapter, we'll look at practical strategies for spreading influence. Recognizing the constraints on our time, these are efficient approaches to building social capital.

7

Practical Strategies for Building Influence

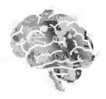

A FEW YEARS AGO, I was traveling to the airport to present at a conference. While briefly stopping by the hospital to check on a postoperative patient, I was called by the operating room. My colleague had a patient on the table and was trying to control the bleeding from a ruptured brain aneurysm—a very high-risk moment. He needed an extra pair of hands. I reflexively ran to the operating room in my nice clean suit and pressed white shirt, feeling worried for my colleague and friend. Together, we saved the patient, just in time.

Once everything stabilized, I felt a nudge against my shoulder: "Man, thanks so much for helping me out. I was losing it there." My usually ice-cool colleague was visibly shaken.

With a grin behind my surgical mask, my response was reflexive. "I know you would've done the same for me."

He had, a couple of years earlier. It was Dr. Stewart, the fellow neurosurgeon who had helped me out with the Hail Mary I shared in chapter 2 of this book.

Cultivate Social Capital

Until that moment with Dr. Stewart, I did not understand the impact of social capital, yet I had it and used it without hesitation. Social capital is a simple concept. Investing in relationships will build social currency in the bank, which can be used when you need a favor. The situation with Dr. Stewart was a large "ask" on a rush basis.

A more routine situation in my world is that a colleague will check on my patients when I am out of town. When my colleagues need to travel, I'll return the favor. Over time, this reciprocity builds more trust than any single favor could.

Building social capital requires influence. Unfortunately, we physicians don't have extra time to invest in relationships. Our time is so overcommitted that we barely have enough time to eat. Building relationships sounds nice, but given our situation, we need savvy, time-efficient approaches. Here are three physician-specific strategies.

Strategy 1: Acknowledge Individual Efforts

Physicians concentrate on the big win; we are high achievers by nature. The downside is that we often do not take time to focus on the everyday small wins. This was a common oversight for me. I have learned over the years that building a team is about creating momentum—and celebrating small wins builds momentum faster than anything else.

Celebrate small wins and anchor the behavior. I recall working with Dr. Kumar, a busy and well-respected gastroenterologist. He complained that the endoscopy suite never started on time and that his whole day was ruined as a result. But Dr. Kumar himself was the problem. Despite his disdain for the "inefficient" schedule, Dr. Kumar rarely arrived early to greet the patient for the procedure. His own failure to prepare often resulted in a twenty-minute delay. He was oblivious to the domino effect his lackadaisical approach would have on not only his start time but also that of the anesthesiologist and support staff.

The administrator spoke with Dr. Kumar regarding his tardiness. After reviewing the call logs and listening to the complaints, the doctor agreed to come in earlier, so that the 7:00 a.m. procedure had a better chance of actually starting on time.

After a week, Dr. Kumar was holding up his end of the bargain. The endoscopy staff playfully created a small scoreboard: "On-time starts: Dr. Kumar 5, Late 0." When I ran into Dr. Kumar in the hallway, he mentioned the scoreboard. I could tell he was amused. The small celebration made him feel good and made it easier to anchor the behavior. The team rarely started late again. I learned that small celebrations make a big impact.

Tell people how they make your day better. Here's another throwback to my neurosurgery training days. Dr. Lorenzo

Muñoz never had a pen when we were doing our rounds in the hospital. Every morning when he came to sign the operative consent forms, he spent minutes looking for a pen. It was frustrating.

Then one day, I watched the beginning of a miracle unfold. Dr. Muñoz was, as usual, looking for a pen when the receptionist handed him one, and he smiled. "Every time you have a pen for me, my day gets better," he told her.

Every day until I left that service, the receptionist had a pen waiting for him.

Years later, I can attest that statement works like a charm. For instance, the front desk receptionist always has a list of my patients ready to hand me when I round on the hospital floors... and don't worry, I always have a pen waiting too.

Compliment a person in front of others. Everyone appreciates compliments. I was coming off a trauma call one morning and the trauma team, the ICU nurses, and I were all gathered around the reception desk. The attending trauma surgeon, Dr. Amos, patiently listened to the flat presentation by the junior surgical resident, Dr. Derrick.

At the end of his presentation, she commented, "Dr. Derrick is a no-nonsense kind of doctor when it comes to excellent patient care."

That compliment in front of a third party was impactful. When Dr. Amos validated Dr. Derrick, complimenting him in front of his peers, she elevated him within the group and also built his social capital. Dr. Amos subconsciously influenced all of us to adopt the complimentary view of Dr. Derrick, regardless of his bland personality.

Remember birthdays. I never really celebrated birthdays, but a few years ago, the neurosurgical ICU changed my opinion on why it's important to mark that moment. It was my birthday, but the day was so busy that I completely forgot. I walked into the unit and the staff gave me a picture of a birthday cake. I was touched that they had remembered me. The nurses said, "We know how you like to watch your carbs, so the real cake"—pointing to the table in the corner—"is for us. This one's for you."

I chuckled and took a big piece of the cake from the table. As I put the fork in my mouth, I said, "Good thing it's my cheat day today."

The birthday cake picture is pinned next to patient letters and cards I keep on a bulletin board. Every time I look at it, I'm reminded of how a group of people made me feel special by just remembering my birthday.

These days, I conscientiously add the birthdays of colleagues to my calendar. And on their birthday, I send a small text. This gesture is a new thing for me. Everyone appreciates a quick "Happy Birthday" text or even a picture of a cake.

Use food to connect. I once overheard a disgruntled surgeon complaining to the operating room charge nurse about the special treatment of other surgeons. The objection was that Dr. Patel was getting special treatment for after-hours staffing. The charge nurse firmly responded that it had nothing to do with policy, but rather that staff volunteered to stay late for Dr. Patel's cases. In the background, one of the nurses jokingly said, "Yeah, it's always pizza night when we do." Apparently, a little pizza goes a long way.

Investing in
relationships
will build social
currency
in the bank.

If the staff stays late to take care of a patient, order pizza for everyone. If you make rounds on the weekend, pick up a box of doughnuts for the staff. This technique is rooted in science. Food causes the brain to release dopamine, and dopamine release causes us to feel pleasure. Teams that feel good about each other have more connection and give each other extra leeway and consideration.

Embrace the power of "we." On the day after my NG tube debacle (see chapter 3), the attending on rounds that morning asked what had happened with the patient, Mr. Stevens, the night before. There were about seven of us: the other surgical residents, a couple of medical students and nurses, and me. The smell of vomit was etched into my brain, so I hesitated before answering.

The chief resident, Dr. Joshua, smoothly covered for me in the pause. "I made a mistake when the NG tube was inserted," he said. "We took care of the issue. The NG tube is now in, and the patient is doing well."

The attending gave us a nod of approval, and we moved on to the next issue.

By taking the blame that day—"*I* made a mistake"—and sharing credit—"*We* took care of the issue"—Dr. Joshua gained my loyalty with the power of "we." He was with me. So I was going to be with him.

Though, of course, "we" all knew what really happened—including the attending physician.

Share your medical cases. In my first year serving in a leadership role, I started a group text with senior physicians. The idea seems pretty intuitive now, but back then it was a novel idea. The text string started out with routine announcements.

The announcements then evolved into a forum—a chat—where physicians could share difficult and unusual cases.

At first, I was reluctant to share cases because, as a young leader, I didn't want to appear incompetent, but I loved it when others presented their "What would you do?" scenarios.

Unexpectedly, when others did share their difficult cases, I found myself developing a greater affinity for them. Their vulnerability and openness led to an unspoken camaraderie, and the group chat became a psychological safe place. The feeling that we were all in this together encouraged me to feel and act the same. What I felt and learned was that empathy connected us through sharing those cases. And that led to improved respect among colleagues.

Strategy 2: Teach Others

Up to this point in the chapter, I have discussed the importance of consistent, small individual efforts and the counterintuitive utility of vulnerability. The second strategy for building alliances is to teach others.

Teaching will build rapport and increase your influence. For busy physicians, teaching is a personal sacrifice. The audience appreciates that selfless time commitment, and that in itself will earn you their respect. The act of teaching also demonstrates that you're interested in other people's welfare and want to give back, and that creates social capital.

In addition, through teaching, you influence a person's ideology and methodology on the subject matter. You will perhaps even create like-minded people—and like-minded people connect more easily.

Teaching in the Intensive Care Unit

Working in the intensive care unit (icu) is complex and can be stressful for a new doctor. When I first started practicing in 2009, I met an intuitively bright nurse in the neurological icu named Stacey. Not long afterward, my colleagues and I were able to convince her to join our neurosurgery practice, and she became the lead nurse practitioner.

Stacey frequently served as the charge nurse in the unit and mentored younger nurses and, nonchalantly, new doctors. The neurosurgeons in the group respected and trusted her. While writing this section, I asked her, "What is the best way for doctors to improve their influence with nurses?"

She smiled and in her Texas twang said, "Dr. Patel, you have one opportunity to make a first impression. Start with friendly and open questions."

Then with her gentle smile, her tone became a little more direct. "Teaching nurses and the other staff members is not a grand rounds 'pimping session' or the Socratic method, where there are rapid-fire questions. Nurses, nursing assistants, and respiratory therapists have been taught to revere the white coat."

She continued without skipping a beat. "They are in a vulnerable position in comparison to a doctor. You need to create a safe space. And that's done by starting with teaching simple concepts. They will then feel safe and be more willing to participate in difficult concepts."

She led me through various icu experiences she had with doctors. Together, we identified three effective teaching methods that can assist doctors in building influence in the icu: informal teaching, formal teaching, and recovery.

Informal teaching. Informal teaching occurs spontaneously while you're diagnosing or performing procedural steps aloud. You will discuss the diagnosis and briefly outline the bedside procedure. This methodology is favored by new and novice nurses because it unfolds in real time. When they understand the relevance and importance of the procedure, and their particular role in it, they are able to take care of the patient better.

Typically, informal teaching involves one or more observing nurses or patient care technicians during a procedure. You will do most of the talking. When posing questions, address the entire group rather than singling out individuals.

Let's walk through a scenario.

Stacey described a time when she was a new nurse and a neurosurgeon placed a bedside ventriculostomy into the brain.

She recalled that the neurosurgeon told the team why the procedure was needed with a simple description: "OK, everyone, I'm placing a ventriculostomy on Mr. Carl because his CT scan demonstrates he has hydrocephalus."

Then the neurosurgeon walked through how and why it was important to them: "I'm moving the head up thirty degrees to decrease pressure in his brain... I'm using lidocaine with epinephrine to not only to numb the scalp but also help with any scalp bleeders..."

Stacey added, "To a new nurse, not only was it fascinating to watch, but also it helped me understand why each step was important and where I needed to help in the future."

"What if having an audience makes me nervous?" I asked.

"If having an audience during a procedure makes you uncomfortable, then I recommend discussing the steps with the nurses *before* the procedure. This will help everyone involved understand your thoughts and next movements."

"Which helps the doctor become less stressed during the procedure," I remarked with a smile.

Formal teaching. Stacey described this as a traditional Power-Point lecture. "Nurses appreciate presentations from doctors. They are rare and help us connect the dots for what matters to you." She stressed that when discussing how to perform a neurological exam, the most effective method is to use a clinical vignette or a typical patient scenario. She concluded by emphasizing, "Remember, simplicity is more effective and inviting."

Recovery. As the conversation progressed, Stacey mentioned a time when a doctor was having trouble performing a lumbar puncture on an ICU patient. During the procedure, the physician became frustrated and became a jerk to everyone in the room. He immediately lost the confidence and respect of the nursing staff due to his behavior, not because of his difficulty with the procedure.

The details of that story sounded a bit too familiar.

Then she told me something unexpected. After the procedure was completed, the remorseful doctor walked over to the nurses, apologized for his behavior, and asked what he could do better next time.

"That insight of owning his poorly handled, stressed-out behavior gained him favor and more respect with the staff." She looked at me with a big smile.

BY SETTING an inviting tone and teaching how the method and science fit together, you influence people to invest in and join your team. No wonder my colleagues were so keen on convincing Stacey to join our neurosurgery practice. She is an invaluable asset to our group and patients.

Giving Back to New Physicians

I used to give mentoring advice by telling young physicians what to do. That was minimally effective. Over the years, I've found the best way to introduce a new idea to a confident but impressionable young surgeon is through the words "I have found that..."

For example, I will say, "Dr. Cho, *I have found that* if I make a vertical incision instead of a horizontal one, the wound heals better." The phrasing makes the information a suggestion in the form of my experience rather than a hard rule that may clash with what Dr. Cho has learned thus far as a resident. The unassuming approach invites young physicians to consider other ideas instead of refusing them by closing their minds.

Teaching as Part of Patient Care

Earlier in this book, I mentioned the Dr. Google phenomenon. Many patients will have done their homework before their clinic appointment. They will arrive at the visit with either a preconceived understanding or complete confusion about their issue. Our job is to lead them toward clarity. The first step to clarity is helping them distinguish between fact, fiction, and the unknown. Sometimes, we may simply have to communicate that there is no single right answer.

Intellectual humility with patients builds trust. A trusting, well-educated patient is an empowered patient—one who is more likely to take their medication and adhere to their treatment regimen.

Patients can also be our best allies and advocates in the community. Taking the time to teach and contextualize is well worth the effort. Build trust. Through trust, we build allies.

Teaching
will build rapport
and increase
your influence.

Teaching Benefits You Too

I improved my personal public speaking skills by teaching nurses. This journey began as informal didactics with nurses regarding patients' cases outside their rooms and eventually moved to a structured framework at nurse lunch-and-learn meetings.

From this experience, I learned the key concept of "knowing your audience." Sharing information was important, but I found that it didn't capture their attention. I needed to fine-tune my message by asking myself, "What's in it for them?" and "Why should they care about what I am saying?"

Once I understood how to make my message relatable to the nurses, I gained the confidence to finesse a message to speak to people from any walk of life. But it all started with teaching. Teaching became an efficient way to build alliances and develop a new skill set.

Strategy 3: Join a Committee

Individual efforts and teaching build relationships without a large time investment. Sometimes, however, we will have to invest time. That brings up the third strategy for building influence—joining a committee.

I strongly encourage you to join an internal hospital committee, medical community organization committee, or local community organization that resonates with you. Yes, these groups do require a time commitment, but they offer numerous benefits both to you and the organization you represent.

A committee membership provides exposure to the layers of an organization. It offers a unique opportunity to shape policies, procedures, and the manner of implementation for patient care. The committee members gain a deeper understanding of the complexity of competing interests at play. You learn to navigate solutions that require the support of other members of the organization. And you are forced to understand how decisions impact not only you but everyone involved.

Drive the change instead of being driven by it.

Build Your Curriculum Vitae

Medical school students and hopefuls strengthen their curriculum vitae (cv) through volunteering and research. As practicing physicians, our cv is built by serving on committees. Committee service demonstrates sacrifice, leadership potential, and cross-disciplinary understanding. These are the things that allow us to be promoted to leadership positions in the real world.

My leadership journey started with the Operating Room Committee. It was within this setting I encountered the tardy Dr. Kumars of the world. Through this experience, I gained insight into the complexities of operating room staffing issues, particularly while managing a physician who voiced constant complaints (see more on how we dealt with Dr. Jay and his tantrums in chapter 10). I became aware of the importance of culture and what it took to keep staff morale high during tough times, which led to much of the advice in this chapter. By serving on a committee, I provided value to the organization beyond just my clinical skills. It opened doors to other diverse roles that might not have otherwise been available to me. And most of all, it was fulfilling.

Develop Negotiation Skills

The committee work process offers physicians a valuable opportunity for growth by fostering respect for the other members' expertise. We are accustomed to giving unilateral instructions to patients and nurses. Working with a team of experts, we develop another entire set of skills.

The committee process compels us to articulate and negotiate our perspectives while seeking to understand those of others. We have to find common ground and the best way to move forward, aligning various points of view.

At one time, I was involved in a frequently frustrating hospital operational issue—patient discharges. Initially, I believed that discharging a patient was accomplished by simply issuing the order to discharge the patient. My committee colleagues were quick to enlighten me that discharge was a complex effort navigated by a team: the physician, the nurse, the social worker, the pharmacy, and the family who would manage the patient when they arrived home. Each person on the list had their own needs and challenges. And each person on the committee negotiated their important role to accomplish the discharge task.

I have found that the true value of serving on the committees is not limited to problem-solving and understanding the needs of specific departments. The real benefit comes from establishing relationships and becoming accustomed to working with influential members across various disciplines, each of whom bring their unique perspectives.

Build Relationships

A committee naturally builds relationships with peers, administrators, and other hospital staff. They come to know you as a person and not just as another ordinary physician.

For example, I think of the now-retired Dr. Oslow. A silver-haired, gentle, and kind physician, he was involved in a case that was reviewed by the quality committee. Ironically, Dr. Oslow had served on that same committee in years past and had helped build the infrastructure that was implemented that day. Many members of the committee had personal experience with Dr. Oslow, knowing him to be not only a conscientious clinician but also a thoughtful person.

Although the case was measured by strict objective metrics, frankly, Dr. Oslow was not. His character, history, and relationships advocated for him without him having to say a single word. In an ambiguous situation, he received the benefit of the doubt. Physicians and administrators across the hospital vouched for him because they knew him from committees.

This is social capital in action—when he needed it most, Dr. Oslow benefited from all the goodwill and respect he had nurtured over many years.

Build Alliances Now

When the rubber hits the road, I believe people will go the extra mile for those who have shown an interest in them. Work alongside people, acknowledge their humanity, build trust and relationships with them, and you will build your support team. Having good connections and building alliances with others exponentially expands your capacity to handle those circumstances.

Similar to Dr. Oslow, you, too, will have a moment of great need in your career, like it or not. Don't wait until it is too late to build the alliances you will need.

Equipped with these efficient and actionable strategies, you will quickly garner social capital. It's time to become granular and learn nuanced personal interactions with your patients and colleagues. These interactions are the key to elevating how people perceive you as a professional.

8

Why You Need to Speak in "People Terms"

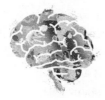

PUSHED THE door halfway open. The room was dim and quiet. The shades were drawn, and a small glow from the table lamp outlined my wife's silhouette. I slowly moved to the far end of the room to a small table hidden in the corner. I sat and waited. I could feel something was wrong. Dread.

"I went to the OB-GYN today," my wife said. "She told me that miscarriage is common. It happens a lot. Then she compared pregnancy to cooking pancakes: 'The first one usually is bad and you throw it out.' I can't believe she compared my pregnancy to a pancake!"

I quickly connected the dots as she continued to speak. The OB had listed facts and statistics, citing my wife's young age among other pertinent factors as to why miscarriage is common. My wife was not comforted.

This was not going to be an easy conversation. I was a young doctor, hadn't become familiar with the situation in my training, and I definitely wasn't familiar with the situation in the present moment. It all felt uneasy and instinctually took me back to the time I spent with Dr. Stone.

Dr. J.R. Stone, a charismatic neurosurgeon, was one of my neurosurgical attendings during my training. He had a distinct, confident stride, and I often imitated him. He stood regally with his hands in his white coat pockets. I, too, held my head high and pulled my shoulders back. I longed for the same air of self-assurance.

By all measures, he was my future self. He was my role model.

One day, Dr. Stone, a small crew of medical students and nurses, and I walked into the neurosurgical ICU to consult on Ms. Swanson. The atmosphere was thick with tension. It was dark and accented by the colorful vital signs on the monitors. Ms. Swanson's family was sitting next to her bed. As we approached, they looked at us with great relief, as if the cavalry had been sent in to save them.

Dr. Stone stood at the end of Ms. Swanson's bed, and after an awkward silence, he cleared his throat and placed his hands in his white coat pockets. And with clinical precision, he delivered the harsh truth: "Ms. Swanson, you did not have a stroke. You have brain cancer."

There was a pause.

"You need a biopsy to confirm the diagnosis. We plan on doing this tomorrow morning."

Yet another pause.

Then Dr. Stone methodically outlined the risks, benefits, and alternatives.

No hope. No faith. No understanding. Just the direct, cold, clinical facts. What I came to understand as "doctor mode."

And there it was, unconsciously etched in my naive and impressionable brain: the methodology for communicating difficult news. Doctor mode.

Doctor mode helped me feel at ease with unfamiliar and emotionally charged situations. It became my default, a lifesaving algorithm, focused and unemotional. Whenever feelings threatened to overwhelm me or I struggled to grasp a situation, doctor mode provided steady ground.

I unconsciously slipped into doctor mode and tried to "fix" my wife through facts and statistics, echoing the debonair Dr. Stone.

"Miscarriages won't affect your future pregnancies; you'll be able to become pregnant again."

"Many women have miscarriages and don't even know it."

"Statistically speaking, a miscarriage likely won't happen again."

But I couldn't "fix" her in that manner. I didn't understand that she needed another form of treatment, one that was neither instinctual nor emphasized in my training.

And here's the truth: How could I understand her? I didn't know how to start. I had never learned.

Up to this point, I had sought and trained my entire career to emulate the heroic Dr. Stone. I had learned to exude his coolness, calmness, and control through my words. And society gave me a nod for that type of communication.

People would say, "Who's your doctor... Dr. Patel? Oh, you're in great hands. He's sincere and direct. Doesn't beat around the bush. You'll appreciate his honesty."

"We trusted his straight talk; no sugarcoating."

The most
important emotional
intelligence skill
is *communication*.

"We didn't know what to believe on the Internet. We needed to know the hard truth. He was calm and matter-of-fact about the possible outcomes. We needed that."

I had successfully carved Dr. Patel in the image of Dr. Stone.

But my wife didn't need me to physically save her life. She needed me to emotionally support her and acknowledge what she had lost. What we'd both lost. She needed me to actively listen and talk through the emotional turmoil—for both of us.

I'd played Dr. Stone for so long that I didn't know how to be anyone else. I didn't have the vocabulary or the skill. Her response to my facts and statistics said it all. She said nothing. And I just sat there not knowing what else to do. That day, two different doctors had failed her.

Here are two things I want you to understand from my experience.

The first is that fixing someone or a situation is not always about eradicating a disease. I wanted to be the heroic doctor. But sometimes the hero needs to just sit in pain with others to ease their suffering—and not through diagnosis and assessment. This is an implied and easily forgotten responsibility of the white coat.

The second thing to take from my experience is that we can prioritize our commitment to mastery of certain skills at the cost of neglecting others. I was forged from the long lonely nights, the countless responsibilities for my patients, and the constant state of mental and physical exhaustion. People expected me to provide stability in an unstable world at a moment's notice. However, adequately carrying out those standards came at a cost.

Dr. Stone was a brilliant neurosurgeon, but he had under-developed communication skills. As an impressionable young doctor, I was eager to learn everything I could from him, even those improper communication skills. In the real world, the emotionally intelligent physician possesses excellent communication skills. Let's look at how to develop the communication that our world needs.

Connect through Communication

As physicians, we are perceived as leaders. And as leaders, we need to be able to connect and influence. Our disadvantage is that we have sacrificed so many years to learning medical terminology, diagnosis, and treatment that speaking in "people terms" was never a priority. However, in the real world, we have to interact with people. Nurses, support staff, and administrators all make decisions that affect us. Building good relationships with all parties—and with other physicians, not to mention patients and their families—makes us better at our calling.

After self-awareness, the most important emotional intelligence skill is *communication*. Successful communication occurs through our words, body language, and actions. The difference between success and failure is not *what* we say, but *how* we say it.

You were smart enough to become a medical student, so I won't cover information on general communication. Feel free to pick that up from any blog or your favorite social media outlet. Instead, I will focus on how communication works in a real-world medical setting, and specifically, the aspects of communication that no one else is teaching you.

The emotionally intelligent, extraordinary physician knows how to connect with others and speak in a way that gets heard. What do the people around you perceive when you speak? What do they think and feel? How can you best communicate your message to them and connect with them? What specific practices are most practical and beneficial?

Communication Is a Dance

Good communication, similar to a good relationship, requires a give-and-take exchange. For example, the friend who only takes—or perhaps only forcefully gives—disrupts the balance needed for a healthy alliance. Communication operates in a similar manner; we must understand how to take cues from the other person and adjust accordingly.

Start with observing the subtleties of body language. If a patient is quiet and not engaged, make the first move to begin a conversation. I suggest asking unscripted icebreaker questions to spark connection and response. (We will discuss exactly how to do this later, in chapter 9.)

In contrast, if a physician colleague is enraged because of the call schedule, their response is unlikely to be mitigated until they feel heard. In that circumstance, it's important to *pause* and *actively listen* to have a worthwhile conversation.

Nonverbal Cues Are Immediate

A few years ago, I was tasked with helping the patient experience team understand why two of our highest-performing surgeons, Dr. Thomas and Dr. Derrick, had received such different scores on their patient satisfaction surveys. Dr. Thomas had scored in the 90th percentile, while Dr. Derrick was below the 50th percentile.

After studying the situation further, we discovered that both surgeons delivered consistently excellent clinical care, but their patients had very different responses to that care. How had this happened?

The patient questionnaires did not demonstrate any obvious revelations at the high level. When we dug deeper into the written comments, however, the trend was striking. Patients responded to Dr. Thomas with warmth. They provided feedback such as:

- "Dr. Thomas makes me comfortable."
- "She listens to me. Easily approachable."
- "She's easy to talk to."

In contrast, Dr. Derrick had a range of responses from patients under his care, for example:

- "Very good doctor, direct and to the point."
- "Serious and knowledgeable."
- "In a hurry."
- "Matter of fact."
- "Distant. I'm not sure he was listening."

Of course, comments never tell the full story, but both physicians were amenable to being observed by a "patient experience educator." The role of this educator was to independently observe and understand ways in which communication with patients could be improved. What obvious differences could she see? What imperceptible cues or impediments could she discern?

Over the next couple of months, we identified a trend that surprised all of us. We discovered that the tone for patient-physician interaction was set within the *first few seconds* of the visit, based on simple social cues. As soon as the educator identified the deficiencies in communication, they seemed obvious. As you can imagine, many physicians consistently overlook them. The cues were simple:

- Offering a welcoming smile
- Humanizing your voice
- Using the patient's name

When a physician used these cues, patients were consistently more satisfied with care. They saw and appreciated the physician's work with clarity.

Even I assumed that I exhibited these cues as if they were second nature. We can discuss my patient experience scores offline. The truth is that we all become tired, distracted, or lost in thought and forget the importance of those first few seconds. If we do, our sincere efforts to help are overshadowed by our "doctor mode" appearance.

To become more conscious of these cues and how and when to use them, let's consider each one more deeply.

Offer a Welcoming Smile

Smiling gives you the biggest bang for your buck. A smile immediately creates warmth and demonstrates interest. It lets the patient know you are happy to help or just to see them. Smiling builds connection and forms the foundation for productive and beneficial communication.

Many of us assume that we are smiling at patients, but heavy caseloads or fatigue can overshadow even our best efforts if we are not intentional. Smiling may appear straightforward, but have you ever observed your own facial expressions when you're rushed or deeply focused on diagnosing a medical condition?

While patients may present with complex medical issues, doctors' focused expressions may not always provide the empathetic connection and reassurance patients are seeking. A smile bridges that gap.

Patients may be high-stakes mysteries, but they're not interested in seeing your poker face.

A "regular" smile is a general facial expression using only the facial muscles. In contrast, a welcoming smile includes the eyes, greets someone warmly, and makes them feel valued.

These days, I usually combine a smile with a slight nod of my head. This creates a welcoming smile through the combination of two nonverbal cues:

- The smile: friendliness and approachability
- The nod: agreement, understanding, and acceptance

The combination of a smile and head nod is a nonverbal way of saying "Hello, I'm glad to see you, and you're welcome here."

The difference
between success
and failure is not
what we say,
but *how* we say it.

Humanize Your Voice

In a pre-mask world, people would kindly tell me, "Doc, your eyes look tired."

In a light-hearted manner, I would reply, "I was born this way" or "I live tired." The joke helped me connect with my patients and let them know my eyes did not accurately reflect my presence. It would soften a flat or distracted tone.

So how can you humanize your voice? Understand that your voice is your verbal personality. Its tone signifies your role. Try to:

- Maintain a calm and soothing tone, avoiding a rushed or overly clinical approach.

- Speak slower, because the patient will perceive a slower pace of speech as thoughtful and more comforting.

- Add a little humor by making fun of yourself.

You know you're superhuman, but patients appreciate it when you humanize yourself with a little humor and a smile in your voice.

Words and How You Say Them

Nonverbal cues are important, but the important part of the communication happens in the actual words said and *how* you say them. A small change in wording can be the difference between a colleague or patient hearing your message or ignoring it. Fortunately, there are easy phrases you can use to help the other person feel heard in a conversation, even if they disagree.

"And," Not "But"

Consider the following example. In the last chapter, I told a story about Dr. Kumar, the well-respected gastroenterologist who had one problem—he was often late. After complaints about the situation reached hospital administration, Dr. Day—the chief medical officer—was tasked with finding a solution. The conversation between Dr. Day and Dr. Kumar went smoothly. Afterward, I asked Dr. Day how he had pulled off that type of cooperation. Dr. Day took a notepad from his desk, leaned toward me, and scribbled.

Approach 1: "Dr. Kumar, yes, we will check our process, *but* we will need to look at your arrival times."

Approach 2: "Dr. Kumar, yes, we will check our process, *and* we will look at your arrival times."

He then directed me to the difference between the emotional tone of these two approaches with very similar wording. The "but" resonated as accusatory, implying Dr. Kumar's guilt. This would have immediately put Dr. Kumar on the defensive, diminishing the likelihood that he would participate in finding a solution. He'd likely respond to any proposed solution as an accusation.

In contrast, saying almost the same line with "and" implied the step was simply another part of the normal process. Accountability was shared. Dr. Kumar would be satisfied (and was) and would listen to the results of the investigation later with an open mind.

Dr. Day then kicked back his chair and propped his cowboy boots on the desk, saying, "And that's how you do it, Dr. Patel." Amazing.

Here are a few more examples of how you might employ an "and, not but" tactic in other common scenarios.

When you are late for clinic duty. "I've waited over an hour for you," a patient accuses.

"Yes, thank you for waiting, *but* we had an emergency that threw off the schedule."

Rather than disputing or downplaying the patient's experience of waiting by using a *but*, we can add to it with a strategically placed *and.*

"Yes, *and* thank you for waiting. We had an emergency that threw off the schedule."

"And" lands with validation of the inconvenience of waiting an hour while giving credit to the words that follow.

In disagreement with a colleague. Use "and," not "but," with a colleague without engaging in a debate.

During a tumor board conference, the medical oncologist stated that the metastatic ovarian cancer patient should have undergone chemotherapy first and then surgery. The gynecology oncologist responded, "Thank you for your comment, *and* we felt surgery would give her the best outcome."

If the gynecology oncologist had responded with "*but* we felt surgery," they would have placed the action in a compromising position, as if their decision required a justification.

To continue goodwill. Imagine walking into the operating room and finding a nicely organized array of surgical instruments ready for your procedure. However, they are not the surgical instruments you typically use. The seasoned operating room technician who set up the table has not worked with you and, therefore, is not familiar with your preferences. Instead of saying, "Thanks, *but* can we set up the surgical instruments I actually use," say, "Thanks, *and* let's also get the surgical instruments I use."

When "and" is used instead of "but," that simple change in one word can balance assertiveness with kindness. "But" implies their efforts were useless, and it's negative and disheartening; "and" allows you to establish future expectations while maintaining goodwill with a person who is vital in assisting your procedure.

Five Phrases

In the same way, using specific words and phrases can help others feel more comfortable and receptive. They can encourage open dialogue. Below are five specific ways to use phrases to validate people without agreeing or disagreeing with them.

Sounds like. A colleague says, "I'm not going to take the COVID vaccine." We can respond, "Sounds like you've made up your mind" without implying agreement or disagreement.

I like that. A surgical team member says, "Nurses should get paid more." We can respond, "I like that."

Makes sense. "Doctors should run hospitals." We can respond, "Makes sense."

Been there. "Parking is terrible here." We can respond, "Yep, been there."

I hear you. "Why are these patients so noncompliant?" We can respond, "I hear you."

These specific words will immediately improve your conversations and relationships.

In the next chapter, I'll continue to offer insights and practical strategies on how to tailor your communication to specific audiences in real-world medical settings.

9

Filling Gaps in Your Communication Training

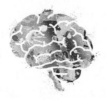

U P TO this point, I have discussed specific techniques to establish connection and choose wording that will be well received. Those skills have little merit if they stand in solitude. If we want to build a productive conversation, we must also be able to listen actively. Active listening requires thoughtful processing with our previously mentioned friend, the prefrontal cortex.

I want to clarify the difference between "active listening" and "hearing." Active listening is a learned skill. That means it must be developed. It requires hearing, brain processing, and then a response. Active listening takes work. On the other hand, hearing is a function, one of the five basic senses. Hearing is passive and not the same thing as active listening.

Without active listening, the back-and-forth dynamic of a strong conversation is broken, and effective communication becomes exponentially harder. Active listening is essential to a conversation.

A few years ago, a colleague, Dr. James, invited me to his office to brainstorm on how to improve patient access to the health system. As I sat across from him at his desk, I noticed his attention intermittently divert downward toward his leg. As our conversation progressed, I realized that his downward gaze wasn't due to shyness. He was texting below his desk— not once, not twice, but repeatedly.

After a moment of disbelief at his discourteous behavior, I politely excused myself from the conversation prematurely. I lost respect for him because of his unprofessionalism and disregarded both the conversation and him altogether thereafter. If he had made any positive points during the twenty minutes we spoke, I couldn't recall them later.

Dr. James undermined his own efforts by not actively listening. To actively listen, he would have needed to stop texting, put down his phone, and make eye contact to engage with me. Had he done so, our project could've started off on the right foot. It's no secret that health care has become fragmented, resulting in siloed patient care communication. Effective communication requires recognition of who is on the other side of the conversation in each instance. This chapter provides guidelines on effectively communicating with patients, nurses, and administrators.

Communication with Patients

Much of our day is dedicated to interacting with patients. While medical school provides *some* basic communication skills, the majority of techniques for effective patient communication are acquired through observing senior residents and attendings. You may have the good fortune to learn from an excellent communicator, or find yourself in the presence of a less notable orator. Unfortunately, the teaching methods can be inconsistent, and successful communication skills are often a matter of chance. The following techniques aim to fill in those gaps and assist you in enhancing spoken communication with patients.

Address Patients by Name

Whenever I meet someone, I consciously take the time to pronounce their name correctly—a rule I made in early childhood.

I remember the first day of third grade. I was so excited. I had my best clothes and new backpack, and all of us would talk about our summer vacation. As the teacher asked us to take our seats, she started a roll call: John Nance, Wendy O'Conner, and... pause.

Embarrassed, I raised my hand. "Yeah, that's me, Nimesh Patel."

I could hear kids in the class giggling. Even I giggled, just to defuse my feeling of awkwardness. As time went on, I even had other teachers pause at my name during roll call and say, "I'm not even going to say *that*." My entire childhood and into adulthood, I anticipated that hesitation to protect my self-worth.

Recently, I was walking through the parking lot and the seven-year-old daughter of a friend said, "Hi, Uncle Nimesh, where's Lana?" She had said my name as if she had said it all her life—a simple gesture that cast light on a shadow that had blotted my entire life to that point. I couldn't believe I had to wait until my forties to be validated by someone other than family in that unexpected moment. I was seen and heard. I was no longer an outcast. And all it took was a little girl's voice.

I cannot emphasize enough how crucial it is to use the patient's name and introduce yourself in return. If you're unsure about how to pronounce their name, simply ask, "What is the best way to say your name?" Always maintain formality by using Mr., Ms., or Mrs., and convey respect for their role as a patient. I typically start with "Hello, I'm Dr. Patel. What is the best way to say your name?"

A personalized introduction goes a long way in establishing intimacy and trust. A name adds a human touch, demonstrating that you see the patient as an individual and care enough to learn their name. You will connect and communicate more smoothly. Learn the nurses' names, too, and, for that matter, lab technicians' names. You should learn every name you can. Knowing a person's name and saying it correctly will make them feel valued and heard, and open them up to you.

Use Unscripted Icebreakers

There are times I have walked into a patient's room full of family members. Even for a veteran physician like me, the sheer number of people in the audience within a confined room can feel intimidating. Here are a few icebreakers aimed at making a good first impression and to establish initial engagement.

- Let's say the patient's last name is Robinson: "Okay, who is Mrs. Robinson in here?" For a crowd, this is by far my favorite question. I find this blanket question warms up the entire room.

- When addressing others in the room, consider asking, "Who do we have here?" This approach, coupled with allowing family members to introduce themselves, helps build rapport and contributes to the patient's decision-making process.

- "Did you find the hospital okay?" "How was traffic?" "How was parking?" These questions are useful even without a family member, and they work by establishing a shared situation with a connection. They also show that you care about their comfort.

Notice how none of these questions is medically related. Each establishes communication with the patient at a non-threatening human level and allows them to relax. A relaxed patient is a key first step to opening up a serious conversation.

Sit or Stand at the Patient's Level

As neurosurgery residents at RUSH, we regularly honed our office clinic skills under the guidance of the esteemed chairman of neurosurgery, Dr. Richard Byrne. Like most neurosurgery residents, I found solace in the operating room. One afternoon, following a fulfilling epilepsy case with Dr. Byrne, I accompanied him to the clinic to assess Mrs. Foster, a fifty-year-old mother of twin boys, who presented with a life-threatening brain tumor.

By this point in my training, I was already a pro at identifying the brain tumor, how to surgically remove it, and what to expect after surgery. Pretty routine stuff. What wasn't routine was the thick awkward silence that followed after Dr. Byrne's confirmation of her life-altering diagnosis.

Dr. Byrne's response in that moment left a lasting impact on my patient communication skills. To break the silence, he adjusted to the patient's level. He pulled out a chair and sat with Mrs. Foster and her husband as I retreated to the corner of the room. He positioned himself to face her, making eye contact. I could sense that his five minutes of parallel sitting were more impactful than my ten minutes standing apart.

Physically matching himself with the Fosters demonstrated he was there with them in spirit, literally at the same level as an equal. By sitting, Dr. Byrne let them know that he was not rushed and that they had his full attention. The simple gesture of meeting them at their level created trust and engagement.

Whenever possible, find a way to sit or stand parallel to a patient's level. It's a simple yet effective way to establish a connection that resonates.

Give Space and Grace

In my first year of practice, Mr. Thomas, a healthy fifty-five-year-old former athlete, visited my clinic for bilateral arm weakness. I attentively listened and documented a detailed history of his complaints, in which he mentioned several

A personalized
introduction
goes a long way
in establishing
intimacy and trust.

times that he had never needed surgery. I continued his assessment by diligently examining the strength and reflexes in his arms and legs. We then reviewed the MRI of his cervical spine together, which demonstrated severe cervical spinal cord compression.

I looked at him and stated, "You need surgery."

As those words left my mouth, I noticed a glaze settle over Mr. Thomas's eyes. It was evident that my subsequent explanations about the surgery duration, hospital stay, and time off work became mere background noise. His attention wavered, drifting away from the conversation at hand.

By the end of our visit, after meticulously walking him through all the procedure details and expectations, Mr. Thomas requested, "Do you mind if I call my wife and have you tell her what you just told me?" Argh. He retrieved his phone, and I found myself repeating the details once more.

When I mentioned this scenario to my senior physician colleagues, they educated me: Mr. Thomas was impacted by a condition called "emotional flooding." When overwhelmed with emotion, patients, like Mr. Thomas, fail to recall information accurately. The phrase "You need surgery" carries significant emotional weight, triggering an adrenaline rush and signaling threat perception in the amygdala, hindering information processing.

Reflecting on this experience, I recognized that I had attempted to deliver a treatment plan prematurely, hindering Mr. Thomas's ability to absorb the information. Consequently, I had to relay the details again to his wife.

Nowadays, I anticipate the glazed stare following the "You need surgery" assessment. I give space by saying, "I can see that the idea of surgery is a lot to think about. Talk to some-one you trust, and come back with questions when you're ready." And have the grace to allow them to invite others into the conversation.

Frame with "Today"

Sometimes, too much conversation can be cumbersome. Dr. Strough was a quirky family practitioner from my hometown, Berea, Kentucky. When I was a kid, he had taken care of my school physicals, occasional strep throat, and rare bouts of poison ivy. He even wrote me a five-hundred-dollar check for a summer *volunteer* job during high school. As a third-year medical student, I returned home for a rural family practice rotation.

Right off the bat, I could see the patients still loved him. The waiting room was crowded, but no one really seemed to mind. However, one afternoon during lunch, Debbie, his practice manager for over twenty-five years, walked into the office kitchen while we were grabbing a quick bite. Without hesitation, she said, "Dr. Strough, our patients have started to notice that you seem a bit rushed during their clinic visits. Some are asking if you're too stressed." Dr. Strough looked at her as if she already knew the answer.

What I learned during that conversation was that the old Dr. Strough had been spending too much time with each patient, and that was costing him in many ways. The new Dr. Strough needed to be more efficient and felt pressured to expedite the visits. In his effort to help all his patients, Dr. Strough's new approach was inadvertently straining his patient relationships.

After studying the issue, Debbie worked with Dr. Strough on a technique designed to maintain momentum in visits while ensuring patients felt heard. She introduced a framing technique called "What brings you in *today*?" For the patients, including "today" subconsciously prioritized their immediate concern.

This allowed Dr. Strough to zero in on the primary issue and redirect the patient, if necessary, by simply asking, "Tell me about today's concern," streamlining the clinic visit. With this technique, patients felt acknowledged, and Dr. Strough smoothly navigated through the visits efficiently.

"Tell me about *today's* concern" has saved many hours in my day.

Summarize and Simplify

There is another important method to ensure your communication with patients is effective and concise.

Mrs. Jones, a lovely seventy-two-year-old woman, was having a tough day. During our clinic appointment, she complained of headaches, neck pain, and back pain, to the point that I began to lose track. I responded, "Mrs. Jones, it sounds like a lot of things are bothering you. Of all these issues, what is the one thing that is bothering you most?"

The "summarize and simplify" technique involves two key steps.

First, summarize what they say out loud. With Mrs. Jones, I first verbalized her concerns back to her, saying, "It sounds like a lot of things are bothering you." This not only confirmed my understanding but also validated her experiences, promoting openness for her to condense her complaints into the core issue.

Second, simplify the complaint. After I summarized Mrs. Jones's feelings, I simplified the complaint—"What is the one thing that is bothering you the most?" This question sets a clear boundary in a friendly way. It takes a diffuse cloud of issues and turns it into a single concern we can solve in the length of a clinic visit. After that, my job is much more manageable.

Team Building with Nurses

While we will speak with patients every day, our conversations with nurses are crucial. Nurses are the lifeline for hospitals and are essential for medical clinics. They are in constant communication with our patients, and that enables them to connect with them and their family members intimately. Nurses help observe and manage patients' emotional and physical pains, which are often hidden and not so readily displayed to physicians. For physicians, nurses' voices can be the difference between a successful case outcome or an unsuccessful one. Nurses will protect the physician and patient when our attention is divided among our many responsibilities. They are worthy of respect for these realities alone. Treat them accordingly.

Ask "Can I Help?"

In my first week as a resident, I watched the nurses preparing to move a patient from a stretcher to the bed. I worked as a

Listening and validating are tremendously important in relationships with colleagues, nurses, and administrators.

certified nursing assistant before medical school, so I was familiar with how challenging this could be, especially with a large patient. The more hands available, the easier the task is for everyone.

I asked, "Can I help?"

The patient was moved, and five minutes later, I went on about my day. I didn't think about it again.

But the nurses and patient care technicians did think about it again. I started to notice subtle lightness and comfort within the stressful environment, and simple things such as a smile that greeted me after a long night, a "Good morning, Dr. Patel" or even a "Busy day, Doc?" Small talk created a more psychologically enjoyable environment. I felt as if I was part of a crew.

Later, after I left that rotation, I discovered a glorious fact. My pager had barely beeped in the middle of the night. In other words, I had been given the precious gift of sleep. Unfortunately, the rumor was that it wasn't the same for my peer residents.

Coincidence? Maybe. Or was it mostly the result of the simple question I asked the nurses: "Can I help?" Three words and probably less than five minutes of pitching in when they needed a hand ended up being a sound investment.

While writing this book, I interviewed Kristin, a nurse colleague. I asked her, "Why are those three words a big deal?"

She chuckled and explained. "Nurses don't typically expect doctors to help. It's not the culture or the protocol."

The fact that I asked "Can I help?" showed that I respected the critical role of nurses on the team. I respected their situation and value, and that elevated me in their eyes.

That willingness of a physician to assist nurses shouldn't be unusual. And yet, somehow, it is. My story is one example of many on how to make the nursing staff our allies. Below are common suggestions from many of the nurses I interviewed. Use them to effectively connect with your nursing team.

Introduce Yourself

When we introduce ourselves, we acknowledge another person's pivotal role and value. It's that simple.

- "Hi, my name is _____."
- I'm on _____ service."
- Smile. (Yes, you know this. But are you doing it?)

Medical students and new physicians rarely introduce themselves to nurses. That's a bad move, as Tu-Vy and Ryan, a couple of experienced charge nurses for our ICUs, described. Tu-Vy told me, "We understand that there are rotations where medical students or residents are here to check the box and leave. You're not interested in the specialty. We get it. But the hospital world is small. We could see you again on another rotation on another floor. You may work here as an attending in a few years, who knows. It costs nothing to be respectful."

She continued, "Introduce yourself and learn other social rituals that grease the wheel of a hospital or clinic."

Other quick phrases to use in a pinch may include:

- "Good morning" or "Good evening."
- "How can I help?"

- "Have a good day!"
- "I know we met earlier. Please remind me of your name?"

My experience has taught me to treat nurses as teammates. Although I may be the "official" authority in the room, including the nurses in the plan makes everyone's lives more pleasant and patient care more effective. Creating a culture of participation shows the nurses that they are valued, as they should be.

Ask to Gain Understanding

In both clinic and hospital settings, the medical field demands continuous teaching and learning. Building rapport with nurses (or senior physicians) is enhanced by engaging them in conversations about their work. Nurses undertake various medical procedures, some of which may be unfamiliar to you. Therefore, don't hesitate to ask.

Reflecting on an earlier incident in this book, a simple question to the nurse could have spared my shoes from vomit. My attempt to insert the NG tube lacked an understanding of nuanced practices.

The next time you find yourself in need of a nurse's assistance, consider using the following script:

- "Hey, Jim, can you help me put an NG tube in on Mr. Stevens? When I saw it done, they curled the tip. What else am I missing?"

- "Mrs. Robinson seems upset about her back surgery. Do you have any insight about why?"

- "Have you seen this before?"

- "Does this look right to you?"

- "Can you show me how you muted the suction alarm?"

- "I've seen this, but I haven't done it yet. Any tips?"

All these questions convey your dedication to learning and improvement, highlighting your commitment despite being new to the field. Every physician started as a new physician. Newness is not incompetency; it's reality.

Succeeding with Administrators

We interact with nurses day in and day out, but it's important to recognize that they're not the only professionals within hospitals or large medical groups. Effective communication with administrators is also vital for becoming a highly successful physician.

I can count on one finger how many times I interacted with a clinic or hospital administrator during my training, and that was because I lost my badge and accidentally walked into the wrong office for a replacement. Times have changed and hopefully interactions have improved, because in the real world, hospital and clinic practice administrators are par for the course.

While preparing for this book, I spoke with several people, one of whom was a new, young liver transplant surgeon. In our conversation, he admitted that the portal vein, vena cava, and aorta didn't make him uneasy—but hospital administrators did. Most likely, this stemmed from his lack of exposure to them.

For such a highly accomplished individual, this surgeon's hesitation around hospital administrators surprised me. He wasn't familiar with their language of strategy, operations, and finance. His unfamiliarity with administrators led him to retreat into a false persona of an arrogant surgeon who spouted complex medical jargon, implying that administrators lacked understanding of patient care complexities. Feeling pigeonholed, he fell into his own stereotype and played the role of the surgeon amplified.

My colleague is definitely not alone. While many physicians easily understand the importance of communicating well with patients and nurses, building a good relationship with an administrator is more challenging.

On the surface, physicians and administrators may appear to have different values. But in my experience, both parties care about patients and economic responsibility, just from different perspectives. The truth is that health care is changing. We must grow, integrating administrators and physicians, or we will not survive.

Make the First Move

Working closely with hospital administrators over the last seven years has given me tremendous insight into how they view physicians. I used to think that they believed in the credo "You do the doctoring, and we'll do the administrating." This myopic view of health care still exists in parts of the United States. However, in my experience, good administrators want to partner with physicians, and together we are looking to improve the lives of our patients.

In researching this book, I interviewed three seasoned health care administrators. Full disclosure: I have worked with all three for years. It has been—and continues to be—a privilege. We have a mutual respect for our commitments to our patients.

I believed that physicians, in general, were reluctant to introduce themselves first, and I wondered if administrators believed the same. To explore this, I posed the same question to all three administrators: "Do you remember a time when a physician introduced themselves to you first? If so, what were your thoughts?"

1 One administrator recounted a physician's transactional interest when introducing himself at a specialty surgical hospital.

2 Another administrator suggested that administrators may be more accustomed to initiating introductions due to frequent business interactions, unlike physicians who typically introduce themselves to patients.

3 A third administrator shared an experience of a physician seeking administrative input to improve connections with medical staff and negotiate a coverage contract, acknowledging the financial aspect of the request.

My takeaway from these conversations was a confirmed belief that physicians rarely take the time to introduce themselves first. And if we do, it's usually for a transactional reason, not out of etiquette.

When I first began practicing, I was hesitant to introduce myself first to administrators because of my lack of previous exposure to them, coupled with an outdated notion of the adversarial us-versus-them relationship. However, in my

There's a greater
upside in asking
"How can I be better?"
than in asking
"How can I get ahead?"

experience, I have found that good administrators want doctors to win. And administrators provide the basic blocking and tackling necessary to move our patients through their journey. In football terms, we have the ball, and they clear the way for us to get into the end zone. Whether in the clinic or the hospital, we need each other to take care of our patients.

Based on my research and personal observations, doctors introducing themselves to administrators first is a novel act. However, by simply doing so, without a complaint or need, you will gain influence and create a favorable relationship.

Ask "How Can I Be Better?"

I consider myself fortunate to have joined a neurosurgery group with supportive mentors who played a pivotal role in my growth. Their guidance was instrumental in my development. By the end of the year, at their encouragement, I called the administrator who had hired me, Paul.

We reviewed the contract to make sure I had met expectations. Toward the end of the call, I asked an off-the-cuff question: "Paul, how can I be better?"

In that moment, everything changed. By the smile in his voice, I realized I had accidentally stumbled onto a golden moment for our relationship.

Fifteen years later, when I caught up with Paul, he still remembered the conversation: "Nimesh, that was the moment I knew you would do well. You were describing how to make yourself invaluable."

All because that one sentence let him know I cared.

If I had postured about my own worth on the phone that day, I would've been one more surgeon in a sea of surgeons.

Rather, when I asked "How can I be better," Paul finished our conversion by recognizing, as he later explained, that I was "someone willing to learn—and to learn from an administrator, a person without a medical degree. We don't get that as often, and therefore you caught my attention."

As medical students and young new doctors, your current success is fueled by competition. Just as mine was. But I encourage you to be mindful that for physicians, the rules in the real world are different. I have learned that there are diminishing returns in the extrinsic philosophy of "How can I get ahead?" Instead, there's a greater upside in asking "How can I be better?"

In the real world, I've discovered that doctors and administrators share more similarities than differences. We both manage stakeholders but in different forms. We both understand the value of working as a team, the importance of collaboration, and the value of structure. While doctors manage clinical decisions that affect patients and families, administrators make health care decisions that affect physicians, nurses, and other medical staff. Both professionals have to consider the broader context and balance multiple interests. Effective communication of decision rationale is essential for successful implementation.

It's All about Relationships

One day, I accompanied Chris, my executive dyad partner, to his tiny office at the hospital. As we reviewed the neuroscience data for the health system, Mr. Carrol, the CEO of the whole system, peeked his head around the door and then plopped his towering six-foot-five frame down on the chair next to me.

What started out as casual banter between two executives and a doctor turned into a deep and thoughtful discussion on the future of neuroscience for the health system. There were things that Mr. Carrol and I both agreed on and a couple of items to which he responded, "I don't disagree. I'm just not there yet. Help me get where you are."

After debating a few more points, he ended the conversation with "Nimesh, when it's all said and done, we can't do this without you all."

With those words, I experienced a sense of validation and understanding that I hadn't actively sought. My intention wasn't to seek validation but to emphasize a point. Our group sought fair compensation for the selfless and unpaid work dedicated to our patients. Mr. Carrol displayed emotional intelligence by recognizing that our primary concern transcended mere economics. In essence, our complaint wasn't about the surface issue but rather a deeper, unconscious matter related to our values. We advocated for principles larger than ourselves and sought acknowledgment for upholding those standards.

That day, I realized the importance of the words "We can't do this without" and how meaningful they were to building a relationship.

Physicians are trained in facts. But with relationships, just face it: facts need to take a back seat to emotion. Validation and connection are key.

As we learned from the doctor mode conversation with my wife that opened chapter 8, diagnosis and assessment can be our default mode of communication—and in many situations, it is ineffective or even detrimental. Look beneath the surface. Listen to patients so you can understand, not just respond with only facts. For that matter, listening and validating are tremendously important in relationships with colleagues, nurses, and administrators as well.

To be clear, a connection is not necessarily about warm fuzzy feelings. Think of the value in building relationships as accumulating social capital. By building trust, we create better workplaces and better working relationships.

Words can help you build influence or destroy it. Use words to build allies and social capital. Put "money in the bank" that you can draw on later. A small amount of effort will pay tremendous dividends in the long run.

Moving on from discussing strategies for tailored communication in medical settings, let's now focus on a crucial skill that separates ordinary practitioners from extraordinary ones—empathy.

10

Empathy Is a Crucial Skill

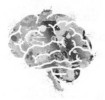

W HEN I was a fifth-year neurosurgery resident, I found myself rushing to the afternoon clinic, which wasn't exactly my favorite part of the job. The sight of the waiting room filled with patients was always overwhelming, to say the least.

Among the crowd that day was Ms. Baker, a respected sixty-year-old businesswoman from our community, accompanied by her husband and her daughter, who happened to be in medical school. Ms. Baker handed me the MRI of her brain, and even at first glance, it was clear she was battling advanced brain cancer.

My mind raced with questions—what could I possibly say about surgery, risks, outcomes, and survival? Despite her understanding of the disease's grim prognosis and her thorough research, she wanted my opinion.

Hardest of all: How do I confirm what she already knows? She is going to die.

Then, unexpectedly, my attending neurosurgeon entered the room. I breathed a sigh of relief. I brought him the MRI images, and he nodded as if he already knew the question that needed to be answered. After a moment of silence, he approached the family and sat down. With a reassuring smile, he told them, "Not on my watch."

In that instant, I felt the weight in the room lift. It dawned on me that Ms. Baker wasn't afraid of death; she feared losing control and dignity. Death was trying to strip away her autonomy. The neurosurgeon's words and, importantly, the confidence and steadiness with which he spoke them assured her that she would not walk alone through this process. He had pledged not to let her suffer; he would unwaveringly stand by her as she battled this disease with clarity and direction.

The surgeon empowered Ms. Baker. He helped her regain her confidence and confront death on her own terms.

SOMETIMES, SURGERY alone isn't enough. Patients and families seek solace not in our medical expertise but in the compassion symbolic of our noble profession.

Ms. Baker's story reveals how empathy can make a difference. Empathy is a silent force, a powerful and understated skill. Can we truly feel someone else's pain, walk in their shoes? I have learned that empathy is not the touchy-feely stereotype I once perceived. It's a powerful skill we have to learn, with time and practice. It's also a soft power that will make you an extraordinary doctor.

Ask about the Patient

Empathy comes to the fore when doctors ask nurses about their patients. The conversation that follows builds a strong bond. It's saying, "Hey, we're in this together." This approach doesn't just improve communication; it makes everyone feel important and responsible for the patient's well-being.

"Nurses love to be asked about their area of expertise, the patient," Judy said with a big smile as we sat in her office. She has been our successful and experienced Methodist Dallas neurosurgical ICU nursing manager for many years. "I often hear from our nurses that medical students and young new physicians are inundated with information on their computer tablets. To understand how the patient is feeling or doing, that information comes most readily from the nurse."

Ask the nurse taking care of the patient, "Do you have any concerns about this patient today?" The simple dialogue changes the relationship with the nurse. It shows that you are colleagues. If an issue or a mistake happens later, the nurse will be more willing to discuss it openly—even if they were the one who made the mistake.

The nurse has information you need. It's wise to ask. Judy continued, "When nurses feel empowered, it makes life easier for both you and them. They become more accountable. Fewer mistakes happen, and the patient receives better care."

Bring the Nurse into Rounds

I'll never forget what the late Dr. Charles Bisig taught me on rounds when I was an eager second-year medical student looking to get into the surgery track. We'd walk the hallways together in between cases. In his surgical cap and with a partly torn surgical mask hanging down on his chest, he said, "Dr. Patel, the nurse is with the patient more than you are. I may not see the patient more than once, but they will. Our patients may not tell us the real issues because they don't want to disappoint us and feel like a burden. But they'll tell the nurses."

He then walked into a patient's room and pushed the call light button. "Hi, this is Dr. Bisig and Dr. Patel. Would you please ask the nurse for Mrs. Jacobs in 5221 to join us in the room, if they are available?"

In that moment, I learned that the simple act of asking the nurse to come into the room with him symbolized to the patient that we all work closely together as a patient care team. It taught me and demonstrated to other staff members—and most of all, to the patient—that Dr. Bisig respected the nurse. That dynamic quickly built trust with patients and families.

Our present-day neurosurgical ICU charge nurse Ryan added, "The nurse will also respect the gesture. If they have information you need, they feel more empowered to ensure an optimal outcome for the patient by relaying any concerns to receptive ears."

I soon saw that this strategy is just plain efficient. One conversation among patients, nurses, and the doctor: communicate the plan to everyone, so doctors and nurses don't have to take time out of their busy schedule for entirely separate conversations.

Empathy is
a silent force, a
powerful and
understated skill.

Dr. Bisig emphasized how important nurses are by always inviting them to join his patient rounds. He displayed empathy once again by acknowledging the nurse's crucial role and promoting collaborative care. By including nurses, Dr. Bisig made sure everyone's ideas were heard. By respecting everyone's expertise, he built trust with patients.

This simple act of working together makes a big difference. Thank you, Chas, my dear friend.

Empathy in All Matters

During my third year in medical school, I shadowed the famous Dr. Jay. He was one of the premier orthopedic surgeons in the state and a physician for the local professional sports team, and his publications were in leading journals. One morning, as I walked in the room to say hello to our first surgical patient, I was surprised to find Dr. Jay at the front desk in the middle of an intense conversation. He was giving the business to some poor soul on the phone. I quickly put the pieces together and learned he was speaking to the hospital president about the lack of staffing in the operating rooms.

Dr. Jay was visibly irritated. He worried that the variability in staffing was putting patients at risk. "These hospital nurses are spread too thin, and this leads to details being dropped. This will eventually hurt a patient." He then slammed the phone down and walked off down the hallway.

During my time on that rotation, I heard Dr. Jay defame the character of the hospital administrators by name. I further learned that this wasn't a new issue. Over the years, he'd complained about the nurses' abilities and alienated the administrators—sometimes even in front of patients. In my eyes, whether or not he was right was immaterial; his emotional outbursts sadly discredited his numerous professional accolades.

After completing that rotation, I found out that an anonymous complaint had been filed against him regarding his lack of professionalism. Ultimately, it was recommended that he have physician behavior counseling to continue practicing. Unfortunately, the staffing issue remained unaddressed.

The lesson I learned from Dr. Jay was to never personalize a problem. The truth was that his concern was an opportunity for improvement. However, because he couldn't channel his anger into a logical argument, he never started a productive conversation on the issue.

Effectively describing an important issue is challenging. It takes self-awareness and emotional intelligence to lay emotions aside. I have heard physicians say, *"You* all didn't hire enough people. *You* didn't plan for this. The failure is on *you."* Instead of using language that guarantees administration will become defensive, use language that invites solutions, such as "How do *we* solve this problem?"

It is true that the squeaky wheel gets the grease. Those who complain do get their concerns addressed faster than those who are quiet. And I am guilty as charged. However, disrespectful tantrums hurt everyone, most of all the profession. In this case, the doctor's personal attacks overshadowed the original issue, and the administrators addressed the seemingly bigger issue—Dr. Jay's behavior.

Dr. Jay's story speaks to the power of empathy in resolving issues. His genuine concern for patient safety was overshadowed by his confrontational behavior, leading to a complaint against his professionalism. If he had taken a more empathetic approach, acknowledging concerns while addressing staffing issues collaboratively, the situation might have been resolved better. Dr. Jay might have polished his reputation instead of tarnishing it, and more importantly, the hospital might have addressed the core issue—the staffing shortages—instead of focusing on disciplining him.

Empathy underscores a distinctive way of speaking and interacting with patients and staff, serving as a cornerstone of our practice.

Now we'll examine nine specific circumstances where silence proves advantageous, drawing from real-world experiences within the health care field.

11

How to Use the Power of Strategic Silence

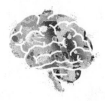

WHEN I first started practicing, one of my more memorable patients, Mrs. Lanai, taught me a lesson I'll never forget.

Mrs. Lanai was an active seventy-five-year-old woman who looked much younger than her age. She told me that over the last few days, her left foot had started to become weak. It now slapped the floor when she walked. (In neurosurgery, we call this a foot drop.)

"I don't understand it. She was doing well until we came home from Hawaii," her concerned husband said.

After another few minutes, I interrupted their story and spoke without hesitation. "Mrs. Lanai, given your age and that foot weakness without any pain, I need to get an MRI of your brain. You may have something up there causing this problem: a brain tumor."

They were stunned, and I spent the rest of the appointment explaining all the facts about a particular benign brain tumor prominent in her age group. I spoke confidently in my assessment, recalling a similar case from my USMLE Step 2 exam in medical school. A tumor compressing a specific part of the brain could cause a painless foot drop, and Mrs. Lanai's description felt like an exact match for the details from my exam.

Two weeks later, Mrs. Lanai returned to the clinic with a CD of her brain images in hand. I looked at the images and flipped through the different sequences. I paused, then looked at the radiology report. I then looked back up at the screen and flipped through her brain images again. There was no brain tumor. The radiologist reported no brain tumor.

I was embarrassed and dismayed. How could I have gotten this so wrong? It was a textbook case.

I took the radical step of asking her to walk me through the events again. "Can you tell me about what happened with your foot, exactly?"

She shrugged. "I was on an overseas flight that day. My legs were crossed for a few hours?"

Oh. I asked specific questions about how she was sitting. This time I actually listened to her answers.

Mrs. Lanai's knee had been pressed against the base of the airplane seat in front of her, a position that had compressed her peroneal nerve. The peroneal nerve travels across the proximal fibula and controls the ability to dorsiflex the foot. Compressing the nerve created the issue. If I'd had a little patience, I would've realized Mrs. Lanai had peroneal palsy, not a brain tumor. Sitting in that specific position had caused temporary nerve damage, which had caused her left foot to drop.

At the follow-up visit, her left foot drop was improving. I prescribed her physical therapy and had her follow up in four weeks.

Mrs. Lanai never had a brain tumor. And I created unnecessary stress for her for two weeks. I'll never get over that. I was too caught up in demonstrating my confidence and competency to notice. I missed the diagnosis because I failed to remain silent.

Instead of showing off my training, I should have listened.

Exercising Silence

Strategic silence is one of the most advanced and influential forms of emotional intelligence. Evolutionarily, we are designed to remain silent—two ears and one mouth. Remaining silent requires us to override our instincts to speak at that particular moment and listen instead. It allows the other person to purge their thoughts and emotions, and to feel heard. Those who speak less often have more influence than those who show their cards by talking.

Let's look at nine specific circumstances under which silence is beneficial. The following tactics are ones I have seen work successfully in the real world of health care.

Tactic 1: Silence to Navigate Relationships with Colleagues
My first venture in leadership consisted of serving on the Multidisciplinary Trauma Peer Review Committee. I enjoyed

the experience because I learned about all the different specialties involved in taking care of a trauma patient. But as months went on, I started to dread those meetings because of Dr. Alan.

Dr. Alan was a stocky trauma surgeon with a big and brash personality. He had joined the health system a few years before me and was not shy about his opinions. Dr. Alan always had to have the last word. Every single meeting, every month. And the problem was, his comments were never-ending. No one knew how to silence him.

One day, Dr. Kennedy also attended the trauma meeting. She was a well-respected senior trauma surgeon. When challenging topics surfaced, I found her comments to be measured and her demeanor internally settled. Her genuine inner confidence was apparent to all in the room, and a welcome contrast to Dr. Alan's more forceful air. With her supportive smile and nods when he spoke, she seemed to understand the angst driving the younger doctor's behavior. Instead of debating him on topics, she'd often remark on his good points and then remain silent. Her poised silence often muzzled Dr. Alan as well.

Amused, I learned that verbal jousting with a last-word colleague only encourages their behavior. Saying nothing and waiting is far more effective. During the committee meetings, Dr. Kennedy showed me how to use strategic silence by validating only the points I agreed with and then continuing supportive, nonconfrontational dialogue through nods and smiles. I now think one layer deeper.

There are times when speaking is the right answer; the key is to know when to speak and when to listen.

Strategic silence
is one of the most
advanced and
influential forms of
emotional intelligence.

Tactic 2: Silence to Build Trust

There is no algorithm to build trust, but there are key moments that build it quickly. When we get these moments right, trust can help us move forward with patient care and colleague collaboration more naturally. Life becomes easier. Strategic silence is highly effective for this purpose.

Very early in my career, Dr. James Moody asked if I would accompany him to visit a patient on whom we would operate together. Dr. Moody observed my presentation of the risks, benefits, and alternatives of the surgery. I provided all sorts of minute details to demonstrate my depth of knowledge on the subject.

We then visited one of his own preoperative patients, and I noticed that Dr. Moody barely spoke. When he did, he asked questions such as "Can you tell me what you understand about the surgery?" and "What concerns do you have about your postoperative pain?" The patient then told him about concerns that I wouldn't have discovered in my standard preoperative visit. Dr. Moody's silence strategically soothed the patient and calmed the environment. The silence created an unspoken trust between Dr. Moody and the patient that encouraged the patient to share their understandings and worries, and it led to a much more efficient and meaningful visit.

Dr. Moody's silence did not indicate a lack of clinical knowledge. He demonstrated that knowledge in a dozen other ways, especially via his emotional intelligence. He smiled at the appropriate times and asked the appropriate questions. Most importantly, though, he knew when to remain silent.

Patients want to share their problems. They want someone to listen. By listening in silence more than speaking, we create trust and learn more about those in our care.

Tactic 3: Silence to Encourage Participation

I have found that it is difficult to convince busy physicians to attend meetings, even ones intended to shape policies that affect them. As a host, I have led meetings with a standard agenda and the opportunity for a Q&A at the end. This format became predictable, boring, and silently optional for my colleagues. If they did attend, they often left early.

One of those colleagues pulled me aside one day and said, "Nimesh, you don't need to take on everything yourself. Learn to delegate. Ask the other physicians to help you."

That's when I decided to strategically stay silent and have the other physicians conduct different sections of the meeting. For a given agenda item, I'd help the physician prepare their speaking points as needed. This delegation of authority led to ownership among the presenters and improved participation by the attendees.

This tactic has worked so well that I rarely conduct any section of the meeting anymore. I just start the meeting with an outline of topics. My goals are far better served by having other physicians run parts of the meeting themselves. Physician involvement and buy-in now feed off each other in a reinforcing cycle.

That's why strategic silence is one of the most effective leadership strategies I know.

Tactic 4: Strategic Silence as a Guardrail

A few months ago, at a meeting about the five strategic initiatives for our health system, a physician started complaining about the quality of food in the physicians' lounge. It was an important concern but not the appropriate forum. And his long rant delayed the discussion of the issues that were actually on the agenda.

The meeting host course corrected the conversation with "I think those are good points, Dr. Alan. Let's talk about that offline, and get through today's agenda." The verbal guardrails politely signaled to Dr. Alan that any topic unrelated to the agenda would be silenced. In this case, the host used "Let's talk about that offline" as a conversation topic boundary. A balance of strategically silencing a tangential conversation with a verbal guardrail is part of good meeting protocol.

Tactic 5: Silence to Get the Job Done

It was a Tuesday at 6:45 a.m. and I stood in front of the operating room reader board studying my surgery case lineup. An anesthesia colleague, Dr. Schafer, walked up to me, bothered.

"Have you heard about the vaccine mandate?"

"I have," I responded cautiously. The government had just mandated the COVID-19 vaccine for all health care providers in the hospital, and there were only a few weeks left before the deadline.

Upset, Dr. Schafer criticized the policy at length. He listed the reasons why he refused to receive the vaccine—all, to me, seemed logical.

However, I found myself wanting to counter Dr. Schafer with additional logical arguments. Then the light bulb went off in my head. By this point in my career, I had seen this kind of situation enough times to understand that the conversation was not about facts. Arguing with him on an emotional topic ran the risk of disrupting our relationship, and likely would make our long workday strained and unpleasant. We had multiple surgeries together that day, and a pleasant working relationship would also positively impact patient care.

So, instead of arguing with him, I practiced pausing. I didn't respond to his argument. When he slowed down to catch his breath, I nodded with validation. "I can see where you're coming from," I said. That's all.

I was ready to retaliate with my own facts. The topic was heated for me as well, but that day, I needed the relationship with Dr. Schafer on a personal and professional level. And risking that for the sake of "winning" would have been poor planning. Instead of fighting for what I wanted, I settled for what I needed.

Tactic 6: Silence to Shift the Power in Your Favor

Most people find negotiations stressful. They are emotionally draining, and for me, they often cause anxiety. From the conversations I have with other doctors, I know I'm not alone. Our training is not in sales, and for most doctors, negotiation is well outside our comfort level. But we live in a world of negotiations. Here, silence can be an amazing tool. Use it to shift the balance of power.

I remember interviewing for my job fifteen years ago. Halfway through the interview, I saw myself at this hospital with this team—the opportunity matched my strengths. When the conversation turned to compensation, the interviewer threw out a number, but not one I was prepared to accept.

By listening in
silence more than
speaking, we create
trust and learn
more about those
in our care.

I had done my homework on compensation for neuro-surgeons. I knew the appropriate number for this particular region, and based on the number introduced by the interviewer, we were not in agreement.

I deliberately said nothing. We just sat there. For more than a minute, the interviewer looked at me and I looked at him, with a thick uncomfortable silence between us.

Finally, the interviewer broke the silence. "Well, what do you think?"

"That's too low," I responded. And my brain said, *Nimesh, did you really just say that?*

His response surprised me; he immediately offered more. He bid against himself.

During the conversation, I felt a power advantage through strategic silence and negotiated more than my researched benchmark. It simply took a moment of silence to generate the result.

This negotiation tactic also works exceptionally well in any situation in which you face an adversary.

Tactic 7: Silence When You Do Not Know the Answer

As physicians, we all encounter a situation when we don't have the answer for a patient. Understandably, this happens more at the beginning of your career. In those moments, remaining silent is an excellent intermediate step.

I mentioned earlier how my predecessor, Dr. Moody, spoke very few words with his patients. He asked a few targeted questions, then switched to listening.

Physicians already receive deference and respect. The patient already assumes you know the answer, even if you don't. Dr. Moody used this: by remaining strategically silent, he allowed the patient to feel confident and to speak freely. The more his patient spoke, the more they felt heard. When the patient expressed questions and concerns that did not pertain to the procedure, Dr. Moody didn't address them, remaining silent instead.

In my fifteen years, I can attest that most of the time, patients are seeking to be heard and understood rather than looking for solutions. You can always look for more answers to their questions later if needed. But silence at the moment buys trust, and that trust buys time and valuable knowledge.

Tactic 8: Silence to Modulate Emotion

Remember the story at the start of this book about the father verbally steamrolling a pediatric oncologist, until Dr. Robinson, the ICU attending (who was also the head of the children's hospital), stepped in? She remained silent while the father continued his angry rant; she listened patiently and did not back down or disagree with him—and he suddenly stopped yelling, slumped into a chair, and burst into tears.

Families crave moments when they can speak with the doctor. Dr. Robinson had one moment to share with that father, and she spent it in silence, listening and engaging with him. She let the father express his emotion, without fighting back. If we can hold our ground and not take the storm personally, our empathetic silence will make the emotion pass quicker.

Tactic 9: Silence for Rest and Recharging

There are moments in our health care journey when we feel utterly alone and drained of energy. Sacrificing personal time, on-call nights with nonstop patient traffic, and patient demands can be truly brutal. I've been there.

Unfortunately, stress and hard work are an inescapable part of our profession. We dedicate our lives to caring for patients, often at a high cost. Feeling overwhelmed and disconnected from the outside world is, to some extent, our reality. Working with patients is an emotional and psychological roller coaster, but I consider it a privilege to be here.

During residency, I found solace in spending time with a group of residents and friends who weren't in the medical field. We'd eat, share meals and laughter, and indulge in reruns of *Chappelle's Show*. One resident always emphasized how exhausted he felt after being on call, reminding us he was "post-call." His persistence earned him the nickname "Post-Call" among the group. "Is Post-Call joining us tonight?" "Hey, Post-Call, can you pick me up around six tonight, or will you be... [chuckle] post-call?"

Among friends, it was all in good humor, but I also took away a valuable lesson. Even when life feels its toughest, don't be "Post-Call." Everyone recognizes the profession is grueling. Lamenting about inherent challenges devalues the sacrifices we've made to pursue this path. Shift the focus from the temporary difficulties to the benefits of an earned lifelong privilege.

I've come to realize that relentless dedication to work yields diminishing returns, especially when I'm emotionally and physically drained. Identifying my threshold and recognizing the limits of my efficiency has been a challenging journey. While I still rise early to maximize my time, I've learned that working harder doesn't always equate to working smarter. Resting and replenishing energy have proved to be a more effective approach.

The science behind brain function has been extensively researched, with numerous studies highlighting the benefits of rest and recharging. Functional MRI brain studies have consistently shown that sleep facilitates the development of nerve connections through neuroplasticity. Interestingly, the greatest growth in new nerve connections occurs during periods of rest and recharging.

Taking time to recharge allows me to step away from the daily grind and engage in introspection. As an extrovert who thrives on social interaction, spending time with others provides comfort, support, and connection. Conversely, for my more introverted side, solitary projects serve as a rejuvenating source of energy and fulfillment.

Feel free to seek out comfort food and comfortable people. I have a small group who add to—rather than subtract from—my life. The key is to find what is comforting for you individually. Whether it's movies, music, or working out, all these activities promote neuroplasticity and bolster cognitive reserve.

During challenging times, inevitable as they may be, prioritizing self-care becomes paramount. It's your responsibility to carve out time to recharge—even when it's difficult—so that you can reap the rewards of your investment.

Resting and recharging isn't just about recuperating; it's a deliberate effort to elevate your capabilities. By working smarter and with equal intensity, I've discovered a newfound efficiency in my approach.

Silence Is a Virtue

It takes an investment of time and energy—sometimes over years—to build good social relationships and accumulate significant social capital. Once we have the social capital, the trick is to hold on to it.

One of the best ways to preserve social capital is the underappreciated essential skill of medicine: being quiet. The best way to keep from bankrupting the social capital we've built is through strategic silence.

Strategic silence is the most important people skill in our repertoire. It'll save us from major regret and creates opportunities. It safeguards our emotional and social capital.

CONCLUSION
Welcome to Reality

_____

AFTER HIGH school graduation, I was lost on how to navigate the path to medical school. I assumed there was an established pre-med major, only to discover there was no such thing.

I chose the University of Kentucky to stay close to home and support the family business. Back then, the university mailed a thick paper catalog and I chose a path that sounded medical: the College of Health Sciences.

People ask, "Didn't you have a high school guidance counselor to help you?" My only experience with our school's guidance counselor was when she pulled me into her office and asked me why students were congregating to fight in the local Walmart parking lot. To which I responded, "I don't know; I have band practice."

On my first day as a college freshman, sporting a new backpack and with a spring in my step, I bounced up the stone steps of the T.H. Morgan building. The lecture hall greeted me with a warm glow from the afternoon sun filtering through the windows. To my surprise, the hall was full of women. Many of them had bags with Greek lettering on them. I wasn't sure what that meant, but I was certain that these college students were easy on the eyes.

Walking over to a seat next to the wall, I caught a glimpse of a smile. Turned out, it was my own reflection in the window. Peter Barris, my first college professor, entered the room. He had long slicked-back brown hair and a manicured beard. His white polo shirt and mid-thigh-length shorts outlined his golden skin and toned muscles. I remember looking down at my own arms in disappointment.

Professor Barris meticulously delineated the course syllabus and expectations. I hung on every word, hoping to glean insights on how to get into med school, but there were none.

At the end of class, I summoned the courage to approach this tanned Greek god and say, "Professor Barris, I want to go to medical school. What are the steps?"

He paused, looked at me with a blank stare of disapproval, and then with terse lips said, "This is the school of PT. Physical therapy is not a stepping stone to medical school. If your desire is medical school, this is not the way. We are here to develop physical therapists."

My smile faded, and the back of my head started to burn. Swallowing hard, I felt a heavy stone in my throat, nodded, and walked off. I had signed up for the wrong major and had no idea how to get into medical school. Welcome to college.

Why is this story important? The first step toward my career, I stumbled, and it was embarrassing. I felt confused, with no guidance, no precut path. Not all of us will have the resources readily available to help guide us through the labyrinth of life. I'm here to tell you that's OK. Sometimes, we will struggle and feel off-balance. Therein lies the key to success. There is a tremendous, unassuming power in traveling uncertain terrain and finding your way back. The setback is a hidden advantage.

My first day at college was a turning point, similar to my desperate phone call to Dr. Von Roenn many years later. In both moments, self-doubt crept in, and I felt directionless. I was forced to look in the mirror of self-awareness, and I discovered ways to overcome these obstacles. Conquering them made me stronger.

Medical school can be overwhelming, and it's common to feel that everyone else has it all figured out. Achieving high scores on the USMLES and completing a residency undoubtedly boosts your sense of readiness. But that alone doesn't guarantee authentic internal confidence and success in the real world. That genuine assurance and accomplishment is what all doctors strive for.

Knowing yourself and being able to connect with others are the greatest skills a doctor can have. Working to achieve these goals will make you a highly successful and fulfilled physician. The hallmark of an extraordinary doctor.

An Evolution

As aspiring physicians, our journey is one of constant evolution. We strive for the best GPA, fill the CV with extracurricular activities, and push through the late nights studying for the MCAT and board scores. After the doors to medical school have opened, we complete a demanding residency and then move into a well-earned career.

Then our career arc plateaus. However, the drive to create, commit, and accomplish never fades; it's an inherent part of our DNA. Perhaps we redirect our focus to other long-awaited achievements: wealth, a family, embracing our new identity. We search for ways to reclaim the time we sacrificed pursuing this great career. But our convictions have not changed. Embedded deep inside each of us is the desire to evolve.

I wrote this book not only to fill the gap between medical school and the real world but also to provide the foundation for the next phase of your career. I know that when you master the skills within these pages, opportunities will fall into your lap—and you will be prepared for them. I've seen it firsthand.

Study these skills diligently until they become second nature. Use them to build a robust practice led by your reputation and word-of-mouth referrals. Strengthen your position as a respected leader, invited to shape the future of health care alongside hospital executives.

Communicate with confidence, and automatically be exposed to professionals in other health care organizations. Build allies and understand the business of health care; this will, in turn, build your influence and pave your way to impact the sector and the next generation of physicians.

The benefits of mastering these skills extend beyond professional growth. They refine you as a partner and family member. And this combination will create a highly successful and fulfilled physician primed for leadership roles that will transform communities.

Do not underestimate your potential. It's possible for you to be a highly successful and fulfilled physician—to be an extraordinary, emotionally intelligent doctor. The skills I share with you in this book have allowed me to carve out this path, filling my white coat to its fullest potential. I believe that you, too, can do the same.

I am optimistic about the future of physicians in medicine. Let's work together to empower each other.

Acknowledgments

MANY PEOPLE were supportive of me as I wrote this book. In particular, I'd like to thank:

Jessie Benitez
The late Chas Bisig Jr.
Stacey Castellanos
Ryan Chang
Judy Cwikla
Kristy Day
Scottie Day
Miguel De Valdenebro
Katherine Dixon
Bill Dudley
Kristen Fehlbaum
Art Herrera
Alex Hughes
Bob Kiser
John McCracken
John Mehall
Jennifer Morton
Esmir Mujkic
Tu-Vy Pham
John Phillips
Liz Rodriguez
Nency Rojas
Namita Saraf
James Scoggin Jr.
Chris Shoup
Scott Steedman
The late Kelvin Von Roenn
Kendra Ward
Veronica Whorton